MEDICAL TERMINOLOGY IN A FLASH!

An Interactive, Flash-Card Approach

Sharon Eagle, RN, MSN

Nursing Educator, Nursing Program
Wenatchee Valley College
Wenatchee, Washington

D1472965

F. A. DAVIS COMPANY • Philadelphia

F. A. Davis Company
1915 Arch Street
Philadelphia, PA 19103
www.fadavis.com

Printed in the United States of America

Last digit indicates print number: 10 9 8 7 6 5 4 3 2

Acquisitions Editor: Andy McPhee
Manager, Content Development: Deborah J. Thorp
Developmental Editor: Kelly Trakalo
Associate Developmental Editor: Melissa Reed
Manager of Art & Design: Carolyn O'Brien
Medical Illustrations: Anne Rains, MS, CMI
Character Illustrations: Chris Reed, www.chrisreedstudio.com

As new scientific information becomes available through basic and clinical research, recommended treatments and drug therapies undergo changes. The author(s) and publisher have done everything possible to make this book accurate, up to date, and in accord with accepted standards at the time of publication. The author(s), editors, and publisher are not responsible for errors or omissions or for consequences from application of the book, and make no warranty, expressed or implied, in regard to the contents of the book. Any practice described in this book should be applied by the reader in accordance with professional standards of care used in regard to the unique circumstances that may apply in each situation. The reader is advised always to check product information (package inserts) for changes and new information regarding dose and contraindications before administering any drug. Caution is especially urged when using new or infrequently ordered drugs.

0-8036-1366-0
9780-8036-1366-9

*To Mom, Brian, Nicole, Brad, and Mel, all of whom
have supported me with unending patience and encouragement.*

To Georgie, who understands what true support looks like.

*To little Gabe and Seth, who came into the world and made me a Grandma
while I was busy writing.*

PREFACE

Have you ever found yourself confused or intimidated by someone who used medical terms you didn't understand? If so, you are not alone. This is a common occurrence. Health-care providers, be they doctors, nurses, therapists or others, tend to get so comfortable with medical terminology that it becomes a natural way for them to speak. Unfortunately, they sometimes forget that the listener may not understand what they are saying. As a result, important information gets lost in the process, and you may walk away wondering what in the world was said.

If you've ever wondered why it sounds like these people are speaking "Greek," it's because they are doing just that. Most medical terms are derived from the Greek or Latin languages. So it's not your imagination. This really is a foreign language. In a sense, once you have mastered medical terminology, you may consider yourself to be bilingual.

As intimidating as medical terminology can be, the happy fact is that anyone can learn to understand and use it. It involves just a few simple steps that will be described in this book.

Let's get started. To begin, there is good news, and there is bad news. Let's deal with the bad news first. The key to developing a good understanding of medical terminology is memorization. It's safe to say that 90% of your work will involve memorizing the meanings of word parts. I won't kid you. This can be a lot of work. Remember, I said this would be *simple*, but I didn't say it would necessarily be *easy*. It will require that you invest a certain amount of time and effort. For some of you, memorization may come easily. If you are one of these lucky few, then you will very likely sail through this course with little difficulty. However if you are one of the many who struggle with memorization, then you may be considering throwing this book into the garbage about now. Before you do that, please allow me to describe a plan that will help you to be successful.

"Hi, I'm Paige. I'm here to help you learn medical terminology."

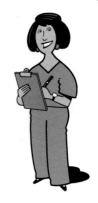

PLAN FOR SUCCESS

Built into this plan are a variety of strategies that will make the task of learning and memorizing word parts much easier.

Textbook

This textbook has many features to support your learning:

- **A narrator, Paige,** leads you through the book and emphasizes many of the key concepts.
- A **workbook format** supports your learning by allowing you to write directly in the book. The act of writing actively engages your brain in a way that reading alone does not. This will enhance your learning.
- **Chapter exercises** allow you to practice translating, creating terms, and using word parts in a variety of ways.
- **An answer key** at the end of the book allows you to check your work. This immediate feedback provides positive reinforcement or immediate correction, either of which will help you learn.
- **Full color anatomical illustrations** of body systems. Body parts are labeled with correct terms, and combining forms are listed. This is reinforced later in each chapter by an exercise that requires you to write in the correct word part associated with each term. This exercise will begin your introduction to human anatomy and will reinforce your association of medical terms to the correct body parts.
- **Color coding of word parts.** You will notice that *prefixes* are coded *green*, **suffixes** are coded **blue**, *combining forms* (word root + a vowel) are coded *teal*, *abbreviations* are coded *orange*, and **pathology terms** are coded **purple**. This color coding directly corresponds with the color-coded flash cards (described below), which may be ordered with this book.

"Be sure to check your answers after you complete each exercise. This helps you learn!"

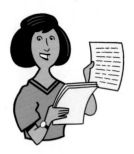

CD Exercises

By completing the fun exercises on the CD-ROM that accompanies this book, you will review medical terms in a variety of ways. Furthermore, you will have the opportunity to practice spelling medical terms, hear terms pronounced, and complete word-building and deciphering exercises.

Flash Cards

Color-coded flash cards that correspond to the word parts in this textbook are available for your use. Most of these cards contain visual cues as well.

- Be sure to practice with the flash cards after you complete each related section of the book. Each day, select a few cards to take with you in your purse or pocket, and review them during otherwise "wasted" moments during the day.
- If you review 5 to 10 different flash cards several times each day in the manner suggested, you can easily memorize 35 to 70 new terms each week without using your "official" study time. Over 10 weeks, that adds up to 350 to 700 new terms! For more ideas on how to use your flash cards, see the following section on Flash Card Games.
- Repetition is the key to memorization; flash cards make repetition easy.
- Because the flash cards are color-coded, you will not only memorize the meanings of the word parts but will also memorize whether the word parts are prefixes, suffixes, combining forms, or pathology terms, without even making a conscious effort!
- The flash cards have terms with the same or similar meanings grouped together. Therefore you will easily memorize two, three, or more terms in the same time it would normally take to memorize just one.

"The key to memorization is repetition. So take some flash cards with you every day."

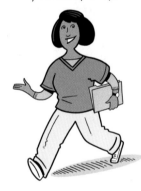

Flash Card Games

- **Partner Flash/2 Players:** Need: 1 set of flash cards. Give selected cards to a partner. The partner will flash each card in front of you, one at a time. You will agree on a preset amount of time to name the correct meaning (5 seconds or less). Run through the cards until you can name each of them within the designated time limit. This is a good exercise to use when your partner does not know medical terminology (such as a family member).
- **Memory Game/1 to 2 Players:** Need: 2 sets of flash cards. Combine 2 sets of flash cards (or selected terms from 2 sets). Shuffle the cards, and lay them out face down in rows. Each partner will take a turn flipping over 2 cards to try to create a "match" (such as two cards that both say "gastro"). In order to get credit for the match, the player must pronounce the term and be able to name the correct English translation (stomach). The player keeps all cards correctly matched and translated. The winner is the player with the most cards at the end of the game. This game can be adapted for just one player. The player simply collects matches one at a time until all cards are used.
- **Speed/2 Players:** Need: At least 6 sets of flash cards. Each partner selects designated cards from 3 sets (such as pathol-

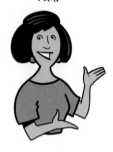

"Flash card games help make learning fun."

ogy terms for the respiratory system). Partners will shuffle their cards and, when ready, will begin laying down cards near each other (each in a separate pile) at the same time. When partners happen to lay down identical cards, the first one to correctly say the term and name the correct definition takes the matching cards from both piles and puts them aside. Matches will be infrequent at the beginning but will occur more and more frequently as cards are eliminated from play. The game continues until all cards are out of play. The winner is the one who collects the most pairs.

- ***Score Four/3 or more Players:*** Need: 1 set per player. Each player contributes a set of designated cards related to one or more body systems. All cards are all shuffled together, and 4 are dealt to each player. Remaining cards are placed in a "draw" pile in the center of the table. The object of the game is to collect all 4 cards of a term. Because the cards have identifying data on both sides, the players will have to hold the cards so that no one else can see them. Players take turns asking one other player for cards with a specific term. For example, Player #1 already has two cards with the term "gastr/o" and wants to collect the other two. On her turn, she may name one other player and ask for all cards with the term "gastr/o." At the same time, Player #1 must correctly pronounce the term and give the correct translation (stomach) in order to "earn" the cards. Player #2 must turn over all cards with that term. If Player #2 does not have that card, then Player #1 must draw a card from the draw pile. Once a player has collected all 4 cards, the player may lay them on the table and must again name the term and the correct translation. If the player forgets these steps when laying down the cards, another player may claim the cards by stating the magic words "Score Four!" and must then pronounce the term and identify the correct translation. If the player is unable to name the correct translation (without looking), the original player keeps control of the cards. The winner of the game is the one with the most 4-card matches when all cards have been played.

ACKNOWLEDGMENTS

To many wonderful people at the F.A. Davis Company I owe a huge debt of gratitude. A heartfelt thanks to Andy McPhee, Acquisitions Editor, for your belief in me and for helping to create the vision. You always seemed to know just when I most needed encouragement and guidance and provided both more times than I can count. Special thanks also to Margaret Biblis, Publisher of Health Professions/Medicine; Melissa Reed, Assistant Editor; Deborah J. Thorp, Content Development Manager; and Kelly Trakalo, freelance developmental editor. I cannot imagine attempting such a huge project without your knowledge and expertise. Others have made their own unique contributions of wisdom, knowledge, energy, and enthusiasm. They include Kimberly Harris, Administrative Assistant; and Kirk Pedrick, Senior Developmental Editor for Electronic Publishing.

Thanks to my students for challenging me with their questions and curiosity and renewing me with their energy and idealism. Ultimately, they are the reason for this book. My hope is that it will serve as a portal into the fascinating world of health care for others like them and provide a good start on a long and rewarding journey.

Finally, my thanks to the reviewers, who took on the time-intensive task of reading through part or all of the manuscript in its various stages and provided valuable feedback and suggestions.

REVIEWERS

Fara C. Amsalem, RN, BSN
Instructor
Allied Health Department
International College
Fort Myers, Florida

Norma Bird, MEd, BS, CMA
Director and Master Instructor, Medical Assisting Program
Health Occupations Department
Idaho State University College of Technology
Pocatello, Idaho

Cori Burns, CMA
Director, Medical Assisting Program
Allied Health Department
Cosumnes River College
Sacramento, California

Christine Cusano, CMA, CPhT
Vice President
Allied Health Department
Clark University
Worcester, Massachusetts

Jeanne Griffith, BS
Director of Training
OIC Training Academy
Barrackville, West Virginia

Tonya Hallock, MA, AS
Director, Medical Assisting Program
Concorde Career Institute
Garden Grove, California

Cathy Kelley-Arney, CMA, MLT-C (ASCP), AS
Institutional Director
Health Care Education
National College of Business & Technology
Bluefield, West Virginia

Joyce Minton, BS, CMA, RMA
Lead Instructor, Medical Assisting Program
Health Sciences Department
Wilkes Community College
Wilkesboro, North Carolina

Lisa S. Nagle, CMA, BSed
Director, Medical Assisting Program
Augusta Technical College
Augusta, Georgia

Vanessa Southard, RN, BSN
Director, Medical Assisting Program
Allied Health Department
New Hampshire Community Technical Colleges
Claremont, New Hampshire

Lori A. Warren, MA, RN, CPC, CCP, CLNC
Co-Director, Medical Department
Spencerian College
Louisville, Kentucky

CONTENTS-AT-A-GLANCE

CONTENTS

INTRODUCTION

LEARNING STYLES

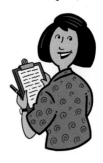

"What's your learning style?"

All people have learning "styles" but no two people are exactly alike. Understanding more about your own unique learning style will aid you in choosing study techniques that will be most effective for you. But how do you identify your style? Read through the descriptions that follow and see which style seems most familiar to you. Most people are actually a combination of styles, but one tends to be dominant.

Solitary Learners

Solitary Learners prefer to study alone. They find the conversation of others to be distracting rather than helpful. They should avoid study groups.

Study Strategies for Solitary Learners

- Find a quiet, isolated place to study, such as a corner of the library or a quiet room in your house.
- Work through all of the exercises in each chapter of this book, and be sure to use the answer key to get immediate correction and feedback.
- Complete the exercises on the CD that correspond to the chapter you are studying.
- Be sure to use the flash cards as directed in the book.
- Select and take 5–10 flash cards with you each day, and review them when time allows. You will get the greatest benefit by using them in the following way:
  — Review them several times, reading the medical term side. Pause and see if you can remember the correct translation on your own. Then flip the card over to see if you are correct.
  — Now review them several more times, reading the English translation side. Pause and see if you remember the correct medical term. Then flip the card over to check yourself.

Social Learners

Social Learners are just the opposite of solitary learners. When they try to study alone, their minds tend to wander, and they are easily distracted. They need to talk with other people and discuss issues in order to "think out loud." Exchanging ideas with others helps them to process the information and gain deeper understanding.

Study Strategies for Social Learners

- Try to identify other social learners in your class with the same needs.
- Make arrangements to study with a partner or in a group.
- Take turns "running" the flash cards with one another.
- Quiz one another using exercises or terms from the book.
- Take turns looking up terms in this book or in your medical dictionary. Practice pronouncing terms and discussing their meanings.
- Persuade family members or roommates to help you by doing some of the same activities described above.
- Be sure to attend class because you need the social interaction. Having the chance to ask questions and participate in discussions will help you immensely.

Auditory Learners

"Auditory learners need to 'think out loud' and hear the spoken word."

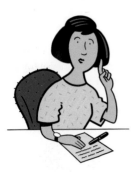

Auditory Learners need to hear the spoken word. When they try to read or study silently, they may notice that their mind wanders. Few people are strong auditory learners, yet nearly everyone can benefit from adding an auditory component to their study techniques.

Study Strategies for Auditory Learners

- Study with others (see suggestions for social learners).
- Listen to others pronounce the terms, and participate in discussions.
- If you must study alone, try reading out loud so that you can listen to your own voice.
- Repeat the terms out loud after you read them or after you hear them. When you first do this, you may feel silly, but you will be amazed at how helpful it is to hear a voice (even your own) speak the terms and translations. Your brain will process and remember the information much better.

- Speak out loud when reviewing the flash cards (for the same reason as described above).
- Listen to the audiotapes. They are extremely helpful in learning the terms and the correct pronunciation.

Be sure to attend class. The class structure provides numerous opportunities to listen to the instructor and classmates pronounce and discuss the medical terms.

Visual Learners

Visual Learners must see the information with their own eyes. Hearing it just isn't enough. For theese people, listening to a dull lecture without the benefit of interesting visuals is equivalent to taking a sleeping pill. They find their mind wandering and cannot understand why they have such a hard time paying attention. Most adults are strong visual learners.

Study Strategies for Visual Learners
- Read this book.
- Take time to review all of the illustrations and tables. It will be time well invested.
- Use the flash cards. They were developed especially for you. Along with the term, they provide a pronunciation guide, strong visual cues, and the English translation.
- The CD-ROM also presents information in a visually appealing manner, so be sure to make full use of it.
- Use colored highlighters on key terms as you read the text. You may even enjoy using highlighters of different colors to "code" or highlight information of different categories.
- Draw pictures, arrows, diagrams, or any other illustrations that help you make connections and understand concepts.

"kinesthetic learners are 'hands-on' people. They learn best by doing it themselves."

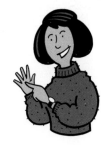

Kinesthetic Learners

Kinesthetic Learners need "hands-on" interaction to learn. Sitting still and listening for long periods drives these people nuts. Observing others is not enough. Kinesthetic learners must *do* for themselves. They can't wait to get up and get moving. They love hands-on activities. Most adults are kinesthetic learners.

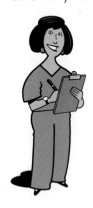

"You may need to try out different techniques to find the ones that work for you."

Study Strategies for Kinesthetic Learners

- You will benefit from many of the same strategies as the social learners. The more interaction you have with others the better.
- Play learning games with the flash cards.
- Completion of learning activities is critically important for you. This includes the book activities, CD exercises and group exercises.
- Attend class so you can do all of the above.

Most adults are predominantly visual/kinesthetic learners, yet possess some of the traits of all of these styles. However you may be the exception. If you are unsure what your style is, try all of these techniques to see what works best for you.

Whatever your learning style, you are sure to find that mastering medical terminology is well worth the effort. Your reward will be the new understanding and insights that you gain. What was once a confusing and mysterious realm will now open it's doors to you. You will begin to understand the language and the world of health and medicine.

MEDICAL WORD ELEMENTS

1

WORD PARTS

Most medical words derive from Greek or Latin and therefore may look and sound odd to you. However, once you have taken the time to learn the meanings of the word parts, you will be able to understand most of the medical terms you encounter, regardless of how big or complex they are.

There are five types of word parts that you need to know. These include: combining forms (created by joining a *word root* to a *combining vowel*), prefixes, suffixes, abbreviations, and pathology terms.

Combining Form

The ***combining form (CF)*** is created by joining a **word root (WR)** with a **combining vowel (CV)**. A **word root** is the main stem of the word. An example using a nonmedical term is the word *walked*. The main stem or root of this word is *walk*.

walked   **CF = WR + CV**

main stem or root word

The purpose of a **combining vowel (CV)** is to make the medical term easier to pronounce. You could say that it makes medical terms more "user-friendly" for the tongue. In nearly all cases, the combining vowel is an **o**, although there are a few exceptions. The combining vowel has no impact on the meaning of the term and is placed between word parts to link them together. For example, consider the root *therm*, which means *heat*. If this word root is combined with an *o* (CV), the result is the **combining form therm/o.**

"The combining vowel does not change the meaning of the word but it does make it easier to pronounce."

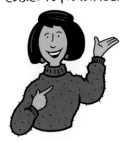

1

When to Use a Combining Vowel

To determine the need for a combining vowel, notice whether the following word part begins with a consonant or a vowel. If it begins with a consonant, as in the word *therm/o/meter*, then a combining vowel (o) is needed. However, if the next word part begins with a vowel (a, e, i, o, u), then no combining vowel is needed. For example, when the word root *arthr*, which means *joint*, is combined with the suffix *itis*, which means *inflammation*, no combining vowel is needed. The term *arthr/itis* is created, which means *inflammation of a joint*. This term may already be familiar to you.

 Pronunciation Tip

When a term is created by using a combining vowel to link two word parts together, the emphasis nearly always shifts to the syllable containing the combining vowel. The vowel (usually an "o") also changes to a short "ah" sound. See the following examples:

thermometer: pronounced thĕr-**MŎM**-ĕ-tĕr

gastroscopy: pronounced găs-**TRŎS**-kō-pē

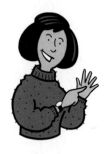

"The prefix comes at the beginning of the word ..."

Prefix

A *prefix* is a word part that comes at the beginning of the word. For example, again consider the word root *therm*. If it is joined with the prefix **hypo** *(beneath or below)* and the suffix *ia (condition)*, then a new word is created: **hypo**/therm/*ia*, a condition of low heat. As you may already know, this term is used in reference to a condition of low **body** temperature.

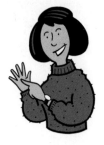

"... and the suffix comes at the end of the word."

Suffix

A *suffix* is a word part that comes at the end of the word. If the suffix **–meter** *(instrument used to measure)* is added to the combining form *therm/o*, the result is the creation of the word *therm/o/***meter**, an instrument used to measure heat.

The terms we have been using are diagramed below so that you can clearly see how the word parts fit together as well as when and why combining vowels are used.

hypo / therm / ia
↑   ↑   ↑
prefix root suffix
(suffix starts with vowel:
no CV needed)

therm / o / meter
↑   ↑   ↑
root   CV suffix
(suffix starts with conso-
nant: CV is needed)

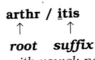

arthr / itis
↑   ↑
root   suffix
(suffix starts with vowel: no CV needed)

Three Simple Steps

There are just three simple steps to follow as you begin decipher-ing medical terms.

1. Translate the *last* word part first.
2. Translate the *first* word part next.
3. Translate *following* word parts in order.

It's that simple. Here is an example. Consider the term **esopha-gogastroduodenoscopy**. This term is quite a mouthful and may seem rather intimidating. However, we will follow the three simple steps described above, and you will see how easy it can be to deci-pher its meaning. You may find it helpful to put slashes between the word parts as demonstrated below. After practicing these steps a few times, you won't need to do this anymore.

esophag/o/gastr/o/duoden/o/scopy

Step 1
–scopy is a **suffix** that means *visual examination*

Step 2
esophag/o is a **combining form** that means *esophagus.*

Step 3
gastr/o is a **combining form** that means *stomach.*
duoden/o is a **combining form** that means *duodenum*, which is the first part of the small intestines.

Now put it all together.
The final translation of esophagogastroduodenoscopy: **visual examination of the esophagus, stomach, and duodenum**, also known as an **upper endoscopy**.

"Translate the last word part.

Now translate the first word part.

Now translate the following word parts."

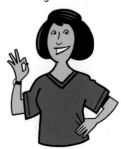

 Memory Tip

It may help you to remember the order in which to complete these steps if you consider the order in which you write your name on most legal documents: *last, first, middle.*

Abbreviations

Abbreviations are used extensively in health care because there are so many terms that are lengthy and difficult to pronounce. Abbreviations save time and simplify the speaking and writing of such terms. Two examples are *CAD*, which stands for *coronary artery disease,* and the large term you just learned, esophagogastroduodenoscopy, which is abbreviated as *EGD*.

Pathology Terms

Pathology terms are used extensively in health care; they refer to diseases and disorders of all body systems. An example is the term **multiple sclerosis**, a chronic disease in which nerves lose the ability to transmit messages to the muscles. Students sometimes struggle with these terms because the three-step deciphering process that you just learned does **not** work with these terms. Learning pathology terms requires memorization. However, this book includes some helpful tips to assist you with this process. The pathology terms are presented in color-coded sections of each chapter and are included in the learning exercises at the end of each chapter. There are also color-coded flash cards for the pathology terms from each chapter.

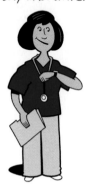

"Abbreviations save time and are much easier to say and write."

CLOSER LOOK

Prefixes

Prefixes are always located at the beginning of a word, and they always modify the meaning of the word in some way. As an example, let's take another look at the word *hypothermia.* The prefix **hypo** means *beneath* or *below.* Therefore, this term indicates a condition of heat that is below normal. A common cause of hypothermia is exposure to cold weather without adequate clothing.

Now let's see what happens when we change the prefix to **hyper**, which means *excessive* or *above.* The newly created word, *hyperthermia*, means a *condition of excessive heat.* This term refers to someone who has a high body temperature. As you can see, changing the prefix can drastically change the meaning of the term. A condition of hyperthermia might refer to a fever caused by an illness such as the flu. Another example is heatstroke, a life-threatening condition caused when a person becomes too hot and dehydrated and does not use adequate cooling measures.

Table 1-1 is a comprehensive list of prefixes for you to memorize. Note that the prefixes are generally arranged in alphabetical order. However, where there are two or more terms with the same or similar meaning, they are grouped together. This will make them easier for you to learn. Don't worry about word building yet. Just focus on learning and memorizing these prefixes. To help you with this process, study Table 1-1 using the following steps.

1. Read the prefixes in the first column.
2. Practice pronouncing the prefix correctly by using the guide in the next column.
3. Read the meaning (out loud) in the second column.
4. Write the prefixes as you pronounce them again (out loud) in the fourth column.

Note that these prefixes will be reviewed again throughout the following chapters.

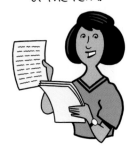

"Prefixes always change the meaning of the term."

TABLE 1-1
PREFIX

Prefix	Pronunciation Guide	Meaning	Write in the Prefix
a-, an-, in-	ā, ăn, ĭn	without, absence of	
ab-	ăb	away from	
ad-	ăd	toward	
anti-	ăn-tē	against	
auto-	aw-tō	self	
bi-	bī	two	
brady-	brăd-ē	slow	
circum-	sĕr-kŭm	around	
dia-, trans-	dī-ă, trăns	through, across	
dys-	dĭs	painful, difficult	
ec-, ecto-	ĕk, ĕk-tō	out, outside	
en-, endo-, intra-	ĕn, ĕn-dō ĭn-tră	within, inner	
epi-	ĕp-ĭ	above, upon	
eu-	ū	good, normal	

(text continues on page 6)

PREFIX *(Continued)*

Prefix	Pronunciation Guide	Meaning	Write in the Prefix
ex-, extra-	ĕks, ĕks-tră	away from, external	
hemi-	hĕm-ē	half	
hyper-, supra-	hī-pĕr soo-pră	excessive, above	
hypo-, sub-, infra-	hī-pō, sŭb ĭn-fră	below, beneath	
inter-	ĭn-tĕr	between	
iso-	ī-sō	same, equal	
mal-	măl	bad, inadequate	
macro-	măk-rō	large	
micro-	mī-krō	small	
multi-	mŭl-tē	many	
poly-	pŏl-ē	much	
neo-	nē-ō	new	
oligo-	ōl-ĭ-gō	deficiency	
para-, peri-	păr-ă, pĕr-ĭ	beside, near	
post-	pōst	after, following	
pre-	prē	before	
pro-	prō	before, forward	
quadri-	kwŏd-rĭ	four	
re-, retro-	rē, rĕt-rō	behind, back	
tachy-	tăk-ē	rapid	
tox-	tŏks	poisonous	
tri-	trī	three	
ultra-	ŭl-tră	beyond	
uni-	ū-nĭ	one	

STOP HERE.
Select the Prefix Flash Cards, and run through them at least 3 times before you continue.

Suffixes

Suffixes are word parts that appear at the end of the word and modify the meaning in some way. Consider the combining form *appendic/o*, which means *appendix*. If the suffix *–itis* (*inflammation*) is added, the term *appendic/itis* is created. As you may already know, this term means *inflammation of the appendix*.

Table 1-2 is a list of suffixes for you to learn and memorize. Note that the suffixes are generally arranged in alphabetical order. However, where there are two or more suffixes with the same or similar meaning, they are grouped together. This will make them easier for you to learn. Don't worry about word building yet. Just focus on learning and memorizing these suffixes. To help you with this process, study Table 1-2 using the following steps:

1. Read the suffixes in the first column.
2. Practice pronouncing the suffixes correctly by using the guide in the next column.
3. Read the meaning (out loud) in the second column.
4. Write the suffixes as you pronounce them again (out loud) in the fourth column.

Note that these suffixes will be reviewed again throughout the following chapters.

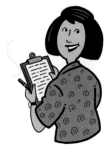

"Suffixes always change the meaning of the term."

TABLE 1-2
SUFFIXES

Suffix	Pronunciation Guide	Meaning	Write in the Suffix
-al, -ac -ar, -ary -ia, -ic -tic* -ical, -ory -eal, -ous, -tous*	ăl, ăk ăr, ār-ē ē-ă, ĭk tĭk ĭ-kăl, ō-rē ē-ăl, ŭs, tŭs	pertaining to	
-algia -dynia	ăl-jē-ă dĭn-ē-ă	pain	
-cele	sēl	hernia	
-centesis	sĕn-tē-sĭs	surgical puncture	
-cide, -cidal	sīd, sĭ-dăl	destroying, killing	
-clast -clasis	klăst klă-sĭs	breaking	

(text continues on page 10)

Suffix	Pronunciation Guide	Meaning	Write in the Suffix
-cyte	sīt	cell	
-derma	dĕr-mă	skin	
-dipsia	dĭp-sē-ă	thirst	
-ectasis	ĕk-tă-sĭs	dilation, expansion	
-ectomy	ĕk-tō-mē	excision, surgical removal	
-edema	ĕ-dē-mă	swelling	
-emia	ē-mē-ă	a condition of the blood	
-emesis	ĕm-ĕ-sĭs	vomiting	
-esthesia	ĕs-thē-zē-ă	sensation	
-gen -genesis	jĕn jĕn-ĕ-sĭs	creating, producing	
-gram	grăm	record	
-graph	grăf	recording instrument	
-graphy	gră-fē	process of recording	
-gravida	grăv-ĭ-dă	pregnant woman	
-ia, -ism	ē-ă, ĭzm	condition	
-iasis	ĭ-ă-sĭs	pathological condition or state	
-ist	ĭst	specialist	
-itis	ī-tĭs	inflammation	
-kinesis -kinesia	kĭ-nē-sĭs kĭ-nē-zē-ă	movement	
-lith	lĭth	stone	
-logist	lō-jĭst	specialist in the study of	
-logy	lō-jē	study of	
-lysis	lĭ-sĭs	destruction of	
-malacia	mă-lā-sē-ă	softening	
-megaly	mĕg-ă-lē	enlargement	
-meter	mĕ-tĕr	instrument for measuring	
-metry	mĕ-trē	measurement	
-oid	oyd	resembling	
-ole, -ule	ōl, ūl	small	
-oma	ō-mă	tumor	

Suffix	Pronunciation Guide	Meaning	Write in the Suffix
-opia	ō-pē-ă	vision	
-osis	ō-sĭs	abnormal condition	
-oxia	ŏk-sē-ă	oxygen	
-paresis	păr-ē-sĭs	slight or partial paralysis	
-pathy	pă-thē	disease	
-pause -stasis	pawz stă-sĭs	cessation, stopping	
-penia	pē-nē-ă	deficiency	
-pepsia	pĕp-sē-ă	digestion	
-pexy	pĕk-sē	surgical fixation	
-phagia -phage	fā-jē-ă fāj	eating, swallowing	
-phasia	fā-zē-ă	speech	
-phobia	fō-bē-ă	fear	
-phoria	fō-rē-ă	feeling	
-plasm -plasia	plăzm plā-zē-ă	formation, growth	
-plasty	plăs-tē	surgical repair	
-plegia	plē-jē-ă	paralysis	
-pnea	pnē-ă	breathing	
-ptosis	tō-sĭs	drooping, prolapse	
-rrhagia -rrhage	ră-jē-ă rĭj	bursting forth	
-rrhaphy	ră-fē	suture, suturing	
-rrhea	rē-ă	flow, discharge	
-rrhexis	rĕk-sĭs	rupture	
-scope	skōp	instrument used to view	
-scopy	skō-pē	visual examination	
-stenosis	stĕ-nō-sĭs	narrowing, stricture	
-stomy	stō-mē	mouthlike opening	
-therapy	thĕr-ă-pē	treatment	
-tome	tōm	cutting instrument	
-tomy	tō-mē	cutting into, incision	
-tripsy	trĭp-sē	crushing	
-trophy	trō-fē	nourishment or growth	
-uria	ū-rē-ă	urine	

*-tic, a variation of -ic is sometimes used; -tous, a variation of -ous is sometimes used

STOP HERE.
Select the Suffix Flash Cards from the deck, and run through them at least 3 times before you continue.

Table 1-3 lists the rules for changing words from the singular to the plural form.

TABLE 1-3				
PLURAL SUFFIXES				
Singular Form	Plural Form	Rule	Singular Example	Plural Example
a	ae	retain the a and add e	vertebra	vertebrae
ax	aces	drop the x and add ces	thorax	thoraces
is	es	drop the is and add es	diagnosis	diagnoses
ix, ex	ices	drop the ix or ex and add ices	appendix	appendices
um	a	drop um and add a	diverticulum	diverticula
us	i	drop us and add i	thrombus	thrombi
y	ies	drop y and add ies	ovary	ovaries

It often takes a considerable amount of practice before the pronunciation of medical terms comes easily and naturally. It will help if you develop good habits right from the start. Carefully review the pronunciation guidelines in Table 1-4. These guidelines will help you learn correct pronunciation.

"Proper pronunciations take practice, practice, practice."

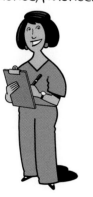

TABLE 1-4		
PRONUNCIATION GUIDE		
Letters	Guidelines	Examples
ps	only the *s* is pronounced	psoriasis (sō-RĪ-ă-sĭs) psychology (sī-KŎL-ō-jē)
pn	only the *n* is pronounced	pneumonia (nū-MŌ-nē-ă) pneumatic (nū-MĂT-ĭk)
g & c	soft sound when used before *e, i,* and *y*	generic (jěn-ĔR-ĭk) gelatin (JĔL-ă-tĭn) cycle (SĪ-kl), cytology (sī-TŎL-ō-jē)

Letters	Guidelines	Examples
g & c	hard sound in front of other letters	gait (gāt) gastric (GĂS-trĭk) caffeine (KĂF-ēn) calcium (KĂL-sē-ŭm)
ae & oe i	pronounced *ē* at the end of a word generally indicates a plural and is pronounced ī or ē	pleurae (PLOO-rē) bronchi (BRŎNG-kī) alveoli (ăl-VĒ-ō-lī)
es	at the end of the word may be pronounced as a separate syllable	nares (NĀ-rēz)

DIRECTIONAL TERMS

Correctly understanding and using directional terms is critical to your ability to accurately communicate descriptive data both verbally and in writing (Fig. 1-1). Table 1-5 provides a list of directional terms.

TABLE 1-5
DIRECTIONAL TERMS

Term	Combining Form	Meaning	Term	Combining Form	Meaning
proximal	proxim/o	nearer to the origin or point of attachment	**distal**	dist/o	further from the origin or point of attachment
medial	medi/o	toward the midline; nearer to the middle	**lateral**	later/o	away from the midline; toward the side
superior	super/o	above or nearer to the head	**inferior**	infer/o	beneath or nearer to the feet
anterior	anter/o	toward or near the front; ventral	**posterior**	poster/o	toward or near the back; dorsal
ventral	ventr/o	front, anterior	**dorsal**	dors/o	back; posterior
deep		further into the body	**superficial**		near the surface of the body
abduction		movement away from the body	**adduction**		movement toward the body

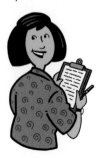

"Don't worry, I've got your dorsum!"

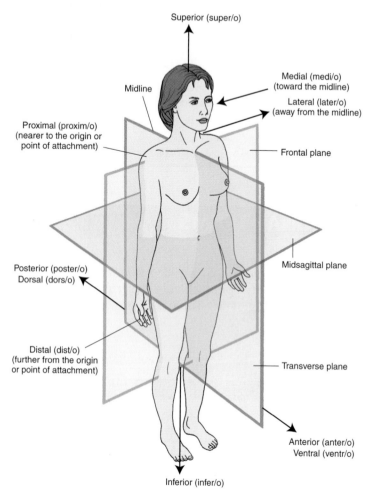

Figure 1-1   Directional terms.

BODY CAVITIES, REGIONS, AND QUADRANTS

The body is divided into a dorsal cavity and a ventral cavity (Fig. 1-2). The dorsal cavity is further divided into the cranial and vertebral cavities. The ventral cavity consists of the thoracic and abdominopelvic cavities.

The nine regions of the abdomen divide it into equal sections, much like a tic-tac-toe grid. The four quadrants divide the abdomen into equal sections, which intersect at the umbilicus (Fig. 1-3).

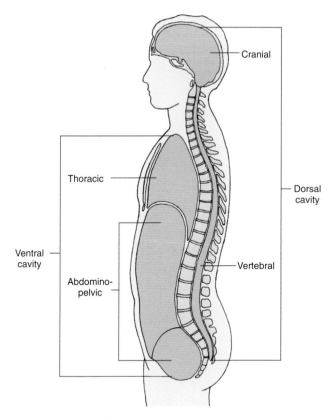

Figure 1-2 Body cavities.

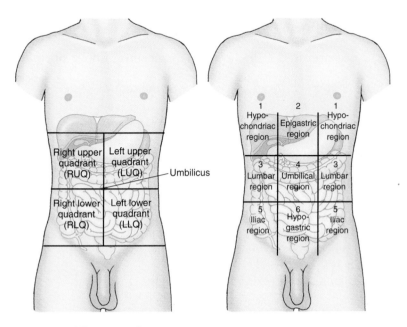

Figure 1-3 Abdominal quadrants and regions.

PRACTICE EXERCISES

Complete the following practice exercises. The answers can be found in Appendix G.

Prefixes

Matching

Match the following prefixes with the correct meanings. Some answers may be used more than once or not at all.

Exercise A

1. _____ tachy-   a. three

"To get the most out of these exercises, be sure to check your answers only AFTER you finished."

2. _____ quadri-   b. half

3. _____ ultra-   c. painful *or* difficult

4. _____ hemi-   d. around

5. _____ hyper-   e. through

6. _____ supra-   f. rapid

7. _____ circum-   g. excessive, above normal

8. _____ dys-   h. same, equal

9. _____ dia-   i. four

10. _____ tri-   j. beyond

Exercise B

1. _____ iso-   a. two

2. _____ a-, an-   b. self

3. _____ mal-   c. new

4. _____ auto-   d. same, equal

5. _____ in-   e. without, absence of

6. _____ ad-   f. below normal, beneath

7. _____ ec-, ecto-   g. bad, inadequate

8. _____ neo-   h. not

9. _____ infra-   i. toward

10. _____ bi-   j. out, outside

True or False

Decide whether the following statements are true or false.

1. True   False   The prefix *retro-* means *back* or *behind.*

2. True   False   The prefix *hypo-* means *below normal* or *beneath.*

3. True   False   The prefix *anti-* means *against.*

4. True   False   The prefix *epi-* means *above* or *upon.*

Fill in the Blank

Fill in the blanks below.

1. The prefix that means *one* is _____.

2. The prefix that means *four* is _____.

3. The prefix that means *small* is _____.

4. The prefixes that mean *beside or near* are _____ and _____.

5. The prefixes that mean *much* or *many* are _____ and _____.

Suffixes

Matching

Match the following suffixes with the correct meanings. Some answers may be used more than once or not at all.

Exercise A

1. _____ -opia	a. digestion
2. _____ -ole	b. urine
3. _____ -scope	c. slight or partial paralysis
4. _____ -pepsia	d. surgical repair
5. _____ -ule	e. breathing
6. _____ -pathy	f. vision
7. _____ -paresis	g. instrument used to view
8. _____ -plasm	h. small
9. _____ -pnea	i. formation, growth
10. _____ -plasia	j. disease

Exercise B

1. _____ -tome	a. incision, cutting into
2. _____ -plasty	b. condition
3. _____ -opsia	c. feeling
4. _____ -phoria	d. surgical repair
5. _____ -tomy	e. disease
6. _____ -phagia	f. vision
7. _____ -uria	g. eating, swallowing

8. _____ -phage   h. growth *or* development

9. _____ -penia   i. cutting instrument

10. _____ -trophy   j. deficiency

11. _____ -ia   k. urine

True or False

Decide whether the following statements are true or false.

1. True   False   The suffix *-pexy* means *surgical fixation.*

2. True   False   The suffix *-pause* means *brief.*

3. True   False   The suffix *-trophy* means *artificial.*

4. True   False   The suffix *-tripsy* means *loosen.*

5. True   False   The suffix *-logist* means *specialist in the study of.*

6. True   False   The suffix *-rrhexis* means *crushing.*

7. True   False   The suffix *-phasia* means *eating* or *swallowing.*

8. True   False   The suffix *-phobia* means *fear.*

9. True   False   The suffix *-rrhaphy* means *suturing.*

10. True   False   The suffix *-scopy* means *stone.*

11. True   False   The suffixes *-cide* and *-cidal* mean *destroying* or *killing.*

12. True   False   The suffixes *-clast* and *-clasis* mean *building.*

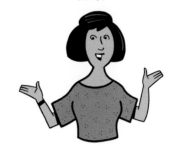

"You're halfway there. Keep up the great work!"

Fill in the Blank

Fill in the blanks below.

1. Suffixes that mean *movement* are _____
   and _____.

2. A suffix that means *record* is _____.

3. A suffix that means *partial or slight paralysis* is

   _____.

4. A suffix that means *mouth or mouthlike opening* is

   _____.

5. A suffix that means *tumor* is _____.

6. A suffix that means *paralysis* is _____.

7. A suffix that means *drooping* or *prolapse* is

   _____.

8. Suffixes that mean *stopping* or *cessation* are
   _____ and _____.

9. A suffix that means *narrowing* or *stricture* is

   _____.

10. A suffix that means *stone* is _____.

11. A suffix that means *surgical puncture* is

    _____.

12. A suffix that means *dilation* or *expansion* is

    _____.

13. List all of the suffixes that mean *pertaining to* _____

    _____.

Directional Terms

1. Fill in the blanks with the correct directional terms.

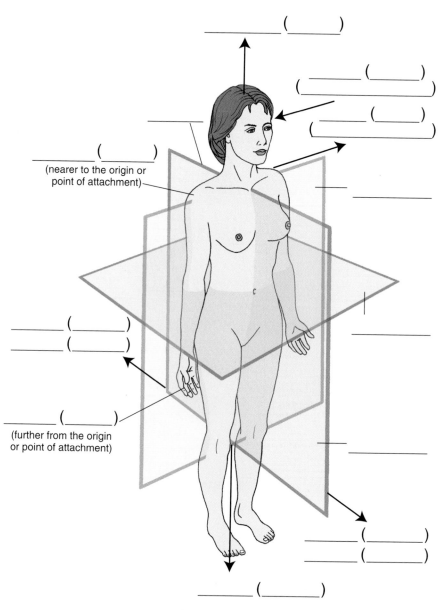

_____ (_____)

_____ (_____)
(_____ (_____)
)
(_____ (_____)
)

_____ (_____)
(nearer to the origin or
point of attachment)

_____

_____ (_____)
_____ (_____)

_____ (_____)
(further from the origin
or point of attachment)

_____

_____ (_____)
_____ (_____)

_____ (_____)

Figure 1-4

2. Fill in the blanks with the correct body cavities.

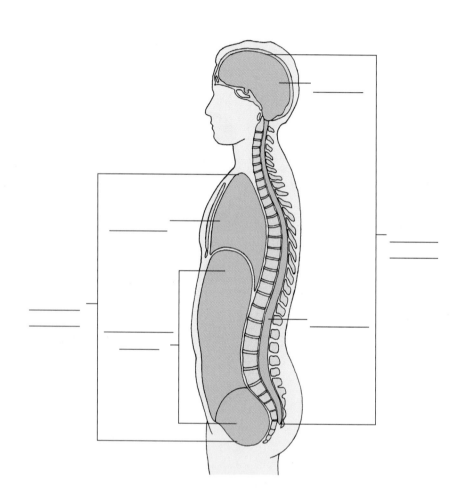

Figure 1-5

3. Fill in the blanks with the correct abdominal regions and quadrants.

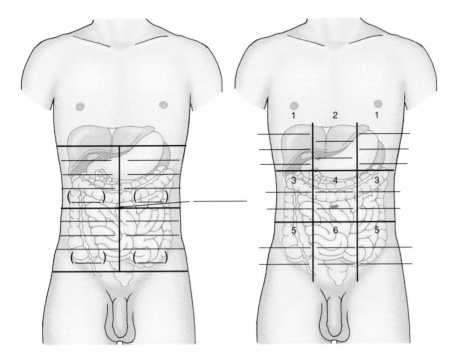

Figure 1-6

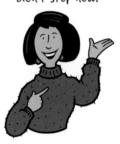

"You're almost done, don't stop now."

Multiple Choice Questions

1. When relating the elbow to the wrist, one might say that the elbow is _____ to the wrist.

   a. proximal

   b. distal

   c. lateral

   d. superior

2. When relating the mouth with the nose, one might say that the mouth is _____ to the nose.

   a. superior

   b. dorsal

   c. proximal

   d. inferior

3. When relating the fingers with the wrist, one might say that the fingers are _____ to the wrist.

   a. superior

   b. medial

   c. distal

   d. anterior

4. The right lung is located _____ to the heart.

   a. anterior

   b. proximal

   c. lateral

   d. ventral

5. Movement away from the body is known as

   a. adduction

   b. abduction

   c. addiction

   d. transverse

Deciphering Terms

Occasionally you will find a word made up of only a prefix and a suffix. Some examples are listed below. Write the correct meaning of these medical terms.

1. bilateral _____

2. diarrhea _____

3. toxic _____

4. unilateral _____

5. hypoxia _____

6. macrophage _____

7. prokinesis _____

8. autograph _____

9. paraplegia _____

10. quadriplegia _____

11. dysphoria _____

12. euphoria _____

13. polyphobia _____

"You did it! Way to go!"

2 INTEGUMENTARY SYSTEM

STRUCTURE AND FUNCTION

You may not think of the skin as an organ, but it is actually the largest organ of the body. The skin consists of three layers (Fig. 2-1). The top layer is the **epidermis.** The epidermis is the thin outer layer that is constructed mostly of nonliving keratinized cells. It is waterproof and provides protection for the deeper layers.

The **dermis** lies just beneath the epidermis and is much thicker. It contains a number of structures, including hair follicles, nerves, blood vessels, and some glands. The base of this layer, aptly named the **basement membrane,** is where new skin cells are produced. These cells are pushed upward as even newer cells form beneath them. Eventually they rise near enough to the top that they die, leaving dry keratinized tissue, and become part of the epidermal layer.

Beneath the dermis is the **subcutaneous** layer. This layer contains fat tissue as well as the deeper blood vessels; nerves; hair follicles, elastin, which provides elasticity; and collagen, which provides strength. The subcutaneous layer provides insulation for deeper structures.

The skin serves several important functions for the body, including protection, insulation, temperature regulation, and blood pressure regulation. Skin protects against bacteria and other microorganisms in several ways. Because the outer layer is waterproof, it doesn't allow organisms entry even when we get wet, unless there is a break in the skin. If microorganisms gain entry through breaks in the skin, such as a **laceration** (cut) or an **abrasion** (scrape), an infection may occur. However, as the tissue becomes irritated, a natural inflammatory response occurs. When this happens, the body increases circulation of blood to the injured area. This is responsible for the signs of **erythema** (redness) and

"epi- is a prefix that means above or upon, so the name epidermis makes perfect sense."

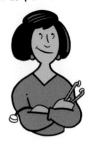

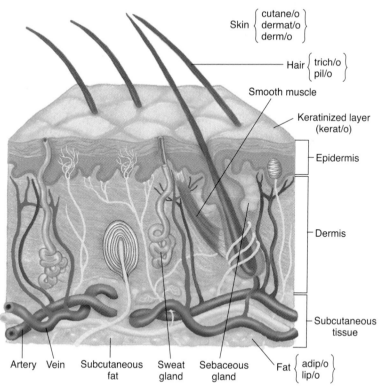

Skin { cutane/o dermat/o derm/o }

Hair { trich/o pil/o }

Smooth muscle

Keratinized layer (kerat/o)

Epidermis

Dermis

Subcutaneous tissue

Artery Vein Subcutaneous fat Sweat gland Sebaceous gland Fat { adip/o lip/o }

Figure 2-1 The skin.

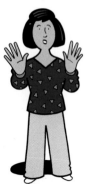

"The skin protects us from outside microorganisms."

edema (swelling) that appear. Increased numbers of **leukocytes** (white blood cells) arrive to fight off the foreign invaders and, quite literally, gobble up the bacteria. The increased blood circulation also helps speed the process of healing as debris is cleared away and healthy new cells and scar tissue fill in the injured area.

The skin contains **melanocytes,** which secrete melanin in response to ultraviolet light from the sun. Melanin is a brown pigment that helps to filter ultraviolet light and protect us from further damage.

The skin also plays an important role in body temperature regulation. It helps to insulate and keep us warm when the external environment is too cold. As this happens, the hands and fingers become pale in color. This is because the blood vessels near the skin surface constrict to give off less heat and conserve the heat for deeper organs. When the environment is too hot, these same blood vessels dilate (expand) in order to give off more heat. This causes a flushed appearance. In addition, the **sweat glands** secrete sweat, which evaporates on the body surface, thus providing even more cooling.

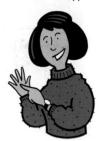

"One, sensory receptors in the skin help to protect us. And, two: sebaceous glands secrete oil to keep our skin soft and supple."

Because the skin contains a number of different specialized **nerves** and **sensory receptors,** it plays a vital role in our ability to perceive hot, cold, pressure, and pain. These messages signal us to take measures to increase our comfort, such as putting on a coat for warmth. In addition, they also provide an important protective function. If you accidentally touch a very hot surface, your heat and pain receptors immediately send a message to your central nervous system (CNS), and you respond by pulling your hand away. This is a protective **reflex,** and it happens so quickly that you don't have time to consciously think about it.

Accessory structures in the skin include the sweat glands, **sebaceous** (oil) glands, **hair,** and **nails.** The hair on our head, eyebrows, eye lashes, nose, and ears serves a protective function as it filters out dust and debris from the air. Nails help to protect the ends of our much-used and often abused fingers and toes. Sweat glands help with cooling. Sebaceous glands secrete an oily substance that lubricates the skin to keep it soft and supple and that also inhibits bacterial growth.

The skin also plays a minor role in blood pressure regulation by dilating or constricting the blood vessels to help raise or lower blood pressure as needed. Blood pressure regulation will be discussed in more depth in Chapter 4.

COMBINING FORMS

Table 2-1 lists the combining forms that pertain to the integumentary system. Table 2-2 lists the combining forms that pertain to color.

TABLE 2-1
COMBINING FORMS

Combining Form	Meaning	Example	Meaning of New Term
adip/o	fat	adipoid (ĂD-ĭ-poyd)	resembling fat
lip/o		lipoma (lĭ-PŌ-mă)	tumor of fat

Combining Form	Meaning	Example	Meaning of New Term
cutane/o	skin	cutaneous (kū-TĀ-nē-ŭs)	pertaining to the skin
dermat/o		dermatologist (dĕr-mă-TŎL-ō-jĭst)	specialist in the study of skin
derm/o		dermoplasty (DĔR-mō-plăs-tē)	surgical repair of the skin
cyt/o	cell	cytology (sī-TŎL-ō-jē)	study of cells
kerat/o	keratinized tissue, cornea	keratotomy (kĕr-ă-TŎT-ō-mē)	incision into the cornea
myc/o	fungus	mycosis (mī-KŌ-sĭs)	abnormal condition of fungus
necr/o	dead	necrosis (nĕ-KRŌ-sĭs)	abnormal condition of dead (tissue)
onych/o	nail	onychomalacia (ŏn-ĭ-kō-mă-LĀ-sē-ă)	softening of the nail
pil/o	hair	pilophobia (pī-lō-FŌ-bē-ă)	fear of hair
trich/o		trichopathy (trĭk-ŎP-ă-thē)	disease of the hair
scler/o	hardening, sclera	sclerosis (sklĕ-RŌ-sĭs)	abnormal condition of hardening
xer/o	dry	xeroderma (zē-rō-DĔR-mă)	dry skin

TABLE 2-2

COMBINING FORMS RELATED TO COLOR

Combining Form	Meaning	Example	Meaning of New Term
albin/o	white	albinism (ĂL-bĭn-ĭzm)	condition of (being) white
leuk/o		leukorrhea (loo-kō-RĒ-ă)	white flow or discharge

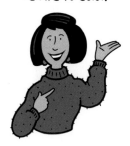

"All of the combining forms in Table 2-2 relate to color."

(text continues on page 28)

COMBINING FORMS RELATED TO COLOR (Continued)

Combining Form	Meaning	Example	Meaning of New Term
cyan/o	blue	cyanosis (sī-ă-NŌ-sĭs)	abnormal condition of blue (color)
erythem/o	red	erythematous (ĕr-ĭ-THĒ-mă-tĭs)	pertaining to red (color)
erythr/o		erythrocyte (ĕ-RĬTH-rō-sīt)	red (blood) cell
melan/o	black	melanoma (mĕl-ă-NŌ-mă)	black tumor
xanth/o	yellow	xanthoderma (zăn-thō-DĔR-mă)	yellow skin

STOP HERE.

Select the Combining Form Flash Cards for Chapter 2, and run through them at least 3 times before you continue.

PRACTICE EXERCISES

Use Tables 2-1 and 2-2 to fill in the answers below.

1. _____ condition of being white

2. _____ yellow skin

3. _____ black tumor

4. _____ abnormal condition of blue (color)

5. _____ white flow or discharge

6. _____ pertaining to red (color)

7. _____ red (blood) cell

8. _____ dry skin

9. _____ resembling fat

10. _____ abnormal condition of hardening

11. _____ tumor of fat

12. _____ fear of hair

13. _____ disease of the hair

14. _____ pertaining to the skin

15. _____ specialist in the study of skin

16. _____ study of cells

17. _____ incision into the cornea

18. _____ surgical repair of the skin

19. _____ abnormal condition of fungus

20. _____ abnormal condition of dead (tissue)

21. _____ softening of the nail

Fill in the blanks with the appropriate combining form.

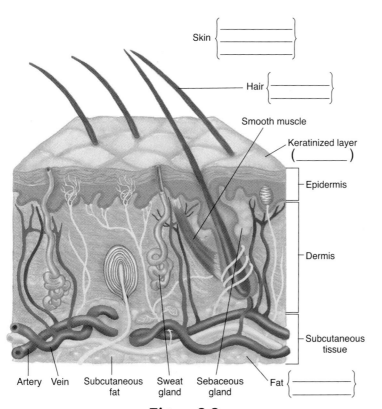

Figure 2-2

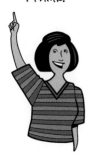

"I can say that term! I think."

ABBREVIATIONS

Abbreviations are used extensively in the world of health care. The primary reason is to save time in both written and verbal communications. As you will see, some medical terms are quite lengthy and difficult to pronounce. This is yet another reason for the use of abbreviations. Imagine having to say **endoscopic retrograde cholangiopancreatography** more than once in a conversation!

Table 2-3 lists some of the most common abbreviations pertaining to the integumentary system as well as some that are commonly used for documentation or medication orders.

TABLE 2-3	
ABBREVIATIONS	
Bx	biopsy
FH	family history
ID	intradermal (injection)
IV	intravenous
I&D	incision and drainage
OTC	over-the-counter
PE	physical examination
SubQ	subcutaneous
Sx	symptom
Tx	treatment

STOP HERE.

Select the Abbreviation Flash Cards for Chapter 2, and run through them at least 3 times before you continue.

PATHOLOGY TERMS

Table 2-4 lists the pathology terms that pertain to the integumentary system.

TABLE 2-4

PATHOLOGY TERMS

abrasion (ă-BRĀ-zhŭn)	scraping away of skin or mucous membranes
alopecia (ăl-ō-PĒ-shē-ă)	absence or loss of hair
cellulitis (sĕl-ū-LĪ-tĭs)	bacterial infection of the skin
comedo (KŎM-ē-dō)	blackhead
cyst (sĭst)	fluid or solid-containing pouch in or under the skin
ecchymosis (ĕk-ĭ-MŌ-sĭs) **contusion** (kŏn-TOO-zhŭn)	discoloration of the skin, a bruise
eczema (ĔK-zĕ-mă)	inflammatory skin disease with redness, itching, and blisters
fissure (FĬSH-ūr)	small cracklike break in the skin (Fig. 2-3A).

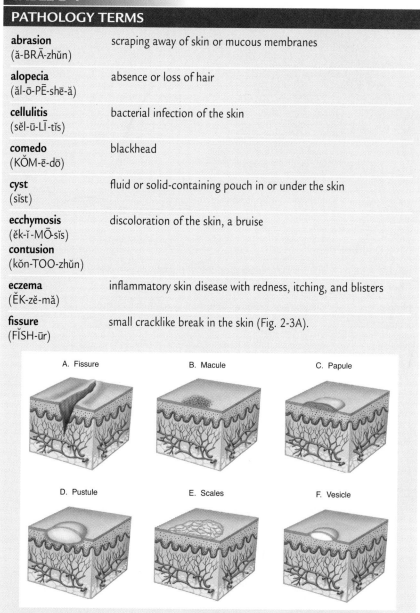

Figure 2-3 Skin lesions. *A,* Fissure. *B,* Macule. *C,* Papule. *D,* Pustule. *E,* Scales. *F,* Vesicle.

(text continues on page 34)

incision (ĭn-SĬZH-ŭn)	surgical cut in the flesh
impetigo (ĭm-pĕ-TĪ-gō)	bacterial skin infection marked by yellow to red weeping, crusted, or pustular lesions; common in children (Fig. 2-4)

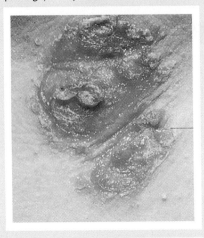

Figure 2-4   Impetigo.

laceration (lăs-ĕ-RĀ-shŭn)	cut or tear in the flesh
macule (MĂK-ūl)	flat, discolored spot on the skin (such as a freckle) (Fig. 2-3B p 31)
papule (PĂP-ūl)	small, raised spot or bump on skin (such as a mole) (Fig. 2-3C p 31)
petechiae (pē-TĒ-kē-ē)	tiny red or purple hemorrhagic spots (Fig. 2-5)

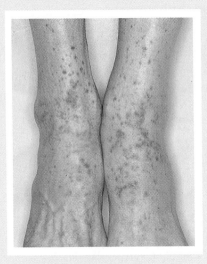

Figure 2-5   Petechiae.
(From Williams LS, Hopper PD: Understanding Medical Surgical Nursing, ed 2. Philadelphia, FA Davis, 2003.)

puncture (PŬNK-chūr)	hole or wound made by a sharp pointed instrument
pustule (PŬS-tūl)	small pus-filled blister (Fig. 2-3D p 31)
scabies (SKĀ-bēz)	contagious skin disease transmitted by the itch mite
scales (skāls)	area of skin that is excessively dry and flaky (Fig. 2-3E p 31)
tinea (TĬN-ē-ă)	fungal skin disease occurring on various parts of the body; also called ringworm or athlete's foot (Fig. 2-6)

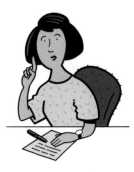

"You may want to refer back to these photos in the clinical area. They're common conditions."

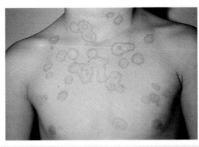

Figure 2-6 Tinea. (From Taber's Cyclopedic Medical Dictionary, ed 20. Philadelphia, FA Davis, 2005, p 2192.)

vesicle (VĚS-ĭ-kl)	clear, fluid-filled blister (Fig. 2-3F p 31)
vitiligo (vĭt-ĭl-Ī-gō)	patchy loss of skin pigmentation (Fig. 2-7)

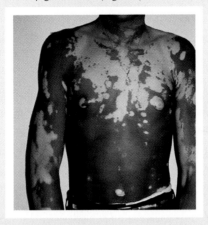

Figure 2-7 Vitiligo. (From Goldsmith LA, Lazarus GS, Tharp MD: Adult and Pediatric Dermatology: A Color Guide to Daignosis and Treatment. Philadelphia, FA Davis, 1997, p 121, with permission.)

STOP HERE.

Select the Pathology Term Flash Cards for Chapter 2, and run through them at least 3 times before you continue.

Memory Tip

The term palpate means "to examine by touch or to feel with your hands." Palpation is one of the methods by which health-care providers examine patients.

Here is an easy way to remember the difference between a *papule* and a *macule:* you can palpate a papule (note that both words start with "p"), but you cannot palpate a macule.

COMMON DIAGNOSTIC TESTS

Allergy testing

Patch test: Paper or gauze saturated with an allergen is applied to the skin. The test result is positive if redness or swelling develops.

Scratch test: Allergens are scratched into the surface of the skin, and the response is noted.

Biopsy: Removal of a tissue sample for microscopic examination.

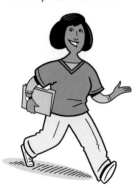

"Here's your first case study. Run with it!"

CASE STUDY

Read the following case study, and answer the questions that follow. Most of the terms are included in this chapter. Refer to the Glossary or to your medical dictionary for the other terms.

Cellulitis

Herbert Marshall is a 56-year-old man admitted to the hospital with a severe case of cellulitis. Mr. Marshall has a history of chronic tinea pedis, which he usually treats with OTC medications. However, when he awoke yesterday, his left foot was erythematous, hot, and tender. He applied an OTC antifungal cream, hoping that would improve his condition. However, today he presented at the clinic complaining of throbbing pain in his foot. The Sx of inflammation have worsened, including increased erythema and edema of the foot and lower leg. After completing a PE, the physician made a diagnosis of cellulitis and admitted Mr. Marshall to the hospital for IV antibiotic Tx.

Cellulitis is an infection of the skin, usually caused when streptococcal or staphylococcal bacteria enter through a break in the skin. Common symptoms include erythema, heat, edema, and tenderness. Treatment for mild cases is oral antibiotics. Severe cases usually require IV antibiotic therapy. Surgical débridement may also be necessary.

Case Study Questions

1. Mr. Marshall's foot has become more
   a. Blue
   b. Red
   c. Dry
   d. Yellow

2. Mr. Marshall's foot has also become
   a. Swollen
   b. Hardened
   c. Bruised
   d. Scaly

3. The physician performed a
   a. Biopsy
   b. Treatment
   c. Physical examination
   d. Incision and drainage

4. Mr. Marshall was admitted to the hospital for
   a. Treatment
   b. A biopsy
   c. Surgery
   d. A subcutaneous injection

5. The antibiotics will be administered to Mr. Marshall by what route?
   a. Subcutaneous injection
   b. Intradermal injection
   c. Intramuscular injection
   d. Intravenous injection

6. Mr. Marshall has a history of chronic
   a. Dry, flaky skin
   b. Blackheads
   c. Loss of skin pigmentation
   d. Athlete's foot

7. The abbreviation Sx stands for
   a. Symptom
   b. Biopsy
   c. Treatment
   d. Injection

(continues on page 36)

8. Cellulitis is usually an infection of the
   a. Hair
   b. Skin
   c. Finger- or toenails
   d. Glands

9. Cellulitis is caused by
   a. A virus
   b. Poor hygiene
   c. Bacteria
   d. Exposure to cold temperatures

10. Cellulitis may be treated by
    a. Oral antibiotics
    b. Intravenous antibiotics
    c. Surgery
    d. All of these

WEB SITES

American Academy of Dermatology: www.aad.org
The Melanoma Research Foundation: www.melanoma.org

PREFIX AND SUFFIX REVIEW

Tables 2-5 and 2-6 contain a review of selected prefixes and suffixes. Refer to these tables as you complete the practice exercises at the end of the chapter.

TABLE 2-5
PREFIX PRONUNCIATIONS AND MEANINGS

Prefix	Pronunciation Guide	Meaning
circum-	sĕr-kŭm	around
epi-	ĕp-ĭ	above, upon, over
hyper-	hī-pĕr	excessive, above
hypo-, sub-	hī-pō, sŭb	below, beneath

TABLE 2-6
SUFFIX PRONUNCIATIONS AND MEANINGS

Suffix	Pronunciation Guide	Meaning
-al, -ic -tic, -ous	ăl, ĭk, tĭk, ŭs	pertaining to
-cyte	sīt	cell
-derma	dĕr-mă	skin
-ectomy	ĕk-tō-mē	excision, surgical removal
-emia	ē-mē-ă	a condition of the blood
-ism	ĭzm	condition
-logy	lō-jē	study of
-lysis	lĭ-sĭs	destruction of
-oid	oyd	resembling
-oma	ō-mă	tumor
-osis	ō-sĭs	abnormal condition
-penia	pē-nē-ă	deficiency
-scopy	skō-pē	visual examination
-trophy	trō-fē	nourishment or growth

PRACTICE EXERCISES

Complete the following practice exercises. The answers can be found in Appendix G.

Matching

Match the following combining forms with the correct meanings. Some answers may be used more than once or not at all.

Exercise A

1. _____ adip/o   a. dry

2. _____ cutane/o   b. fungus

3. _____ derm/o   c. hair

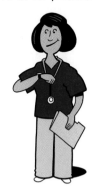

"Time for practice."

4. _____ kerat/o   **d.** keratinized tissue or cornea

5. _____ necr/o   **e.** fat

6. _____ xer/o   **f.** red

7. _____ scler/o   **g.** dead

8. _____ lip/o   **h.** hardening

9. _____ dermat/o   **i.** white

10. _____ myc/o   **j.** skin

Exercise B

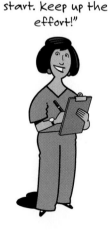

"You're off to a great start. Keep up the effort!"

1. _____ xanth/o   **a.** hair

2. _____ erythr/o   **b.** blue

3. _____ cyan/o   **c.** fat

4. _____ albin/o   **d.** cell

5. _____ trich/o   **e.** fungus

6. _____ onych/o   **f.** red

7. _____ cyt/o   **g.** skin

8. _____ erythem/o   **h.** nail

9. _____ melan/o   **i.** white

10. _____ leuk/o   **j.** black

11. _____ pil/o   **k.** yellow

Word Building

*Using **only** the word parts in the lists provided, create medical terms with the indicated meanings.*

Prefixes	Combining Forms	Suffixes
circum-	adip/o	-al
epi-	albin/o	-cyte
hypo-	dermat/o	-derma
	derm/o	-ectomy
	erythr/o	-emia
	cyan/o	-ic
	cyt/o	-ism
	kerat/o	-oid
	leuk/o	-oma
	lip/o	-osis
	melan/o	-penia
	myc/o	-tic
	necr/o	
	or/o	
	onych/o	
	trich/o	
	scler/o	
	xanth/o	
	xer/o	

1. resembling fat _____

2. pertaining to dry skin _____

3. a condition of (being) white _____

4. abnormal condition of yellow (color) _____

5. pertaining to the skin _____

6. pertaining to above or upon the skin _____

7. abnormal condition of skin fungus _____

8. deficiency of red (blood) cells _____

9. abnormal condition of blue (color) around
   the mouth _____

10. hardening of the skin _____

11. abnormal condition of hair fungus _____

12. abnormal condition of keratinized
    tissue _____

13. white (condition of) blood _____

14. abnormal condition of nail fungus _____

15. black tumor _____

16. pertaining to death _____

17. pertaining to beneath the skin _____

18. surgical removal of fat _____

19. fat cell _____

20. dry skin _____

Deciphering Terms

Write the correct translation of the following medical terms.

1. cyanoderma _____

2. sclerotic _____

3. hyperkeratosis _____

4. leukocytopenia _____

5. hypodermic _____

6. erythrocyte _____

7. dermatology _____

8. melanocyte _____

9. trichomycosis _____

10. hypertrophy _____

11. xeroderma _____

12. xanthoma _____

13. lipolysis _____

14. adiposis _____

15. onychoma _____

16. necrosis _____

True or False

Decide whether the following statements are true or false.

1. True   False   With a **patch allergy test,** a piece of paper or gauze is saturated with an allergen and applied to the skin.

2. True   False   With a **patch allergy test,** the results are negative if redness or swelling develops.

3. True   False   With a **scratch allergy test,** allergens are scratched into the surface of the skin, and the response is noted.

4. True   False   A **biopsy** involves the removal of a tissue sample for microscopic examination.

5. True   False   The abbreviation for **biopsy** is BSY.

6. True   False   The abbreviation **ID** stands for incision and drainage.

7. True   False   The abbreviation for **physical examination** is Px.

8. True   False   The abbreviation **Tx** stands for treatment.

9. True   False   The abbreviation **FH** stands for family history.

10. True   False   The abbreviation **SubQ** stands for sclerosis.

11. True   False   The abbreviation **OTC** stands for over-the-counter.

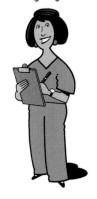

"You learn by repetition, so keep going."

Fill in the Blank

Fill in the blanks below.

1. A term that means *scraping away of skin* is

   _____.

2. Terms that means *discoloration of the skin* or *a bruise* are

   _____ and _____.

3. A term that means *tiny hemorrhagic spot* is

   _____.

4. _____ is a skin infection marked by yellow to red crusted or pustular lesions.

5. _____ causes patchy loss of skin pigmentation.

6. A _____ is a clear, fluid-filled lesion, such as a blister.

7. A _____ is a small pus-filled blister.

8. The medical name for a blackhead is

   _____.

9. _____ is a contagious skin disease transmitted by the itch mite.

10. A small raised spot or bump such as a wart is a

    _____.

11. _____ results in loss of body hair.

12. A _____ is a cut or tear in the flesh.

13. A _____ is a small cracklike break in the skin.

14. _____ is an inflammatory skin disease that causes redness, itching, and blisters.

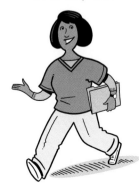

"You're almost to the finish line. Don't stop now!"

15. A _____ is a flat discolored spot on the skin, such as a freckle.

16. A bacterial infection of the skin is called

   _____.

17. The medical name for a fungal infection of the skin commonly known as ringworm is _____.

18. _____ describes an area of the skin that is excessively dry and flaky.

19. A _____ is a solid or fluid-containing pouch in or under the skin.

Common Diagnostic Tests

Write the definition of the following diagnostic tests.

1. **Patch allergy test**

2. **Scratch allergy test**

3. **Biopsy**

Multiple Choice Questions

Select the best answer to the following multiple choice questions.

1. Which of the following terms is **NOT** paired with the correct meaning?

   a. erythr/o: red

   b. xanth/o: white

   c. melan/o: black

   d. cyan/o: blue

2. Which of the following abbreviations is **NOT** paired with the correct meaning?

   a. Bx: biopsy

   b. Tx: treatment

   c. PE: physical examination

   d. FH: history and physical

3. Which of the following pathology terms is **NOT** paired with the correct meaning?

   a. abrasion: scraping away of skin or mucous membranes

   b. contusion: bruise

   c. macule: small, raised spot or bump on the skin

   d. cellulitis: bacterial skin infection

4. Which of the following pathology terms is **NOT** paired with the correct meaning?

   a. comedo: blackhead

   b. cyst: fluid or solid-containing pouch in or under the skin

   c. pustule: small pus-filled blister

   d. fissure: surgical cut in the flesh

5. Which of the following pathology terms is **NOT** paired with the correct meaning?

   a. eczema: inflammatory skin disease with redness, itching, and blisters

   b. scabies: contagious skin disease transmitted by the itch mite

   c. impetigo: patchy loss of skin pigmentation

   d. tinea: any fungal skin disease occurring on various parts of the body

"You've completed the whole chapter. You're a real winner!"

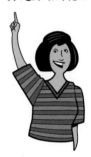

3

NERVOUS SYSTEM

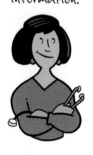

STRUCTURE AND FUNCTION

The nervous system plays a key role in maintaining **homeostasis,** the state of equilibrium in the body. More complex than the most high-tech computer, the nervous system is capable of storing vast amounts of data as well as receiving and sending thousands of messages throughout the body instantly and simultaneously. The nervous system is divided into two parts, the ***central nervous system (CNS)*** and the ***peripheral nervous system (PNS).***

The CNS includes the brain and spinal cord (Fig. 3-1). The brain is where data storage and information processing occurs. The spinal cord is composed of nerves and extends from the base of the brain down to the second lumbar vertebra.

The PNS includes 31 pairs of spinal nerves that branch off from either side of the spinal cord and the nerves in the arms and legs.

 Memory Tip

Remember that the ***central*** nervous system (brain and the spinal cord) is located in the center or most ***central*** part of the body. The ***peripheral*** nervous system is located ***peripheral*** to, or ***outside*** of, the CNS and includes the nerves on either side of the spinal cord and in the arms and legs.

The PNS consists of **sensory** and **motor neurons** (nerve cells). Sensory nerves gather information from the external environment and note things like air temperature. They also note your response to the environment, such as the sensation of discomfort from feeling cold. This information is sent to the brain. The brain responds to this new information by sending messages back out to the body via the motor nerves. The message may be a conscious one that tells your body to move and put on a sweater or it may be an unconscious message such as yawning or breathing faster and deeper to meet your body's need for more oxygen.

"Sensory nerves gather information by sensing changes. Motor nerves tell us to move or respond in some way."

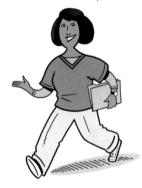

A. Brain

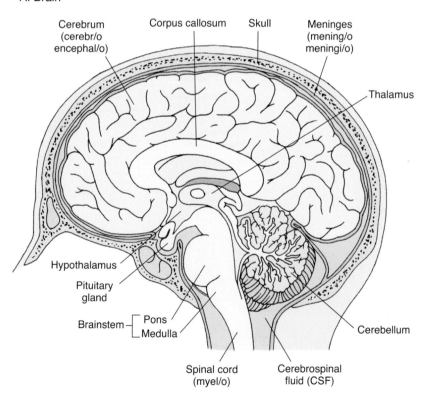

Figure 3-1 The central nervous system. *A*, The brain.

B. Spinal cord

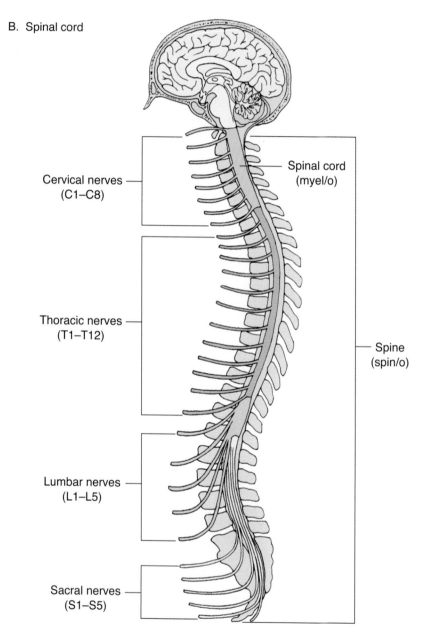

Cervical nerves
(C1–C8)

Spinal cord
(myel/o)

Thoracic nerves
(T1–T12)

Spine
(spin/o)

Lumbar nerves
(L1–L5)

Sacral nerves
(S1–S5)

Figure 3-1   (Continued) *B*, The spinal cord.

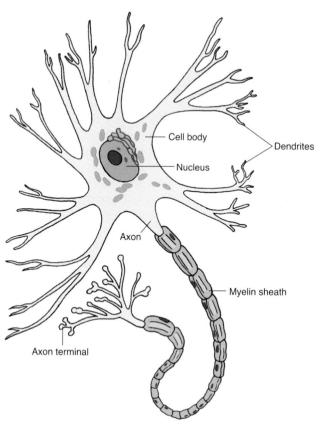

Cell body

Nucleus

Dendrites

Axon

Myelin sheath

Axon terminal

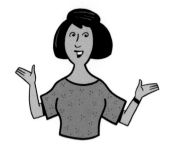

"Human nerve cells are somewhat like very complex extension cords."

Figure 3-2   The neuron.

Figure 3-2 illustrates a nerve cell, known as a **neuron.** Neurons vary in size and shape and have the following key parts: **cell body, axon,** and **dendrites**. The cell body houses all of the microscopic structures that keep the cell energized and functioning. The dendrites, which resemble the branches of a tree, are responsible for gathering information from the internal and external environment and sending this information to the cell body.

The nerve cell in the human body functions in a way somewhat similar to that of an electrical cord that might be found in your home. In an electrical cord, the wires are protected by a rubber coating of insulation. The axon of the nerve cell also has a protective layer of insulation **(myelin)** made from specialized cells. The electric cord sends electricity from the energy source to the refrigerator, television, or other device so that it can operate. The

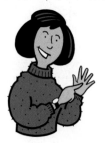

"The brain is protected by the skull, the meninges, and the cerebrospinal fluid."

human nerve cell sends electrical impulses down the axon to muscles, organs, or other tissues in the periphery so that they can function. When the insulating layer of an electrical extension cord becomes frayed or otherwise damaged, the cord may "short out." As a result, signal transmission may be temporarily or permanently lost, and the device no longer works. Similarly, if the myelin layer on the axon degenerates or is damaged, the electrical impulse may be temporarily or permanently lost. As a result, the organ or muscle that it innervates may not function properly. This explains some of the symptoms caused by degenerative neuromuscular diseases such as **multiple sclerosis.**

The brain and spinal cord are protected by several structures. The brain is enclosed and protected by the hard bones of the skull, known as the **cranium,** and the spinal cord is protected by the vertebral column. Protecting both the brain and the spinal cord are three membranes called the **meninges.** Enclosed within the meninges is the cerebrospinal fluid, which circulates continuously to cushion and bathe the brain and spinal cord.

COMBINING FORMS

Table 3-1 contains combining forms that pertain to the nervous system along with examples of terms that utilize the combining form and a pronunciation guide. Read out loud to yourself as you move from left to right across the table. Be sure to use the pronunciation guide so that you can learn to say the terms correctly.

TABLE 3-1
COMBINING FORMS RELATED TO THE NERVOUS SYSTEM

Combining Form	Meaning	Example	Meaning of New Term
cerebr/o	brain	cerebrovascular (sĕr-ĕ-brō-VĂS-kū-lăr	pertaining to brain and vessels
encephal/o		encephalocele (ĕn-SĔF-ă-lō-sēl)	herniation of the brain
gli/o	glue or gluelike	glioma (glī-Ō-mă)	gluelike tumor

Combining Form	Meaning	Example	Meaning of New Term
mening/o	meninges	meningitis (měn-ĭn-JĪ-tĭs)	inflammation of the meninges
meningi/o		meningioma měn-ĭn-jē-Ō-mă	a tumor of the meninges
myel/o	spinal cord, bone marrow	myelography (mī-ĕ-LŎG-ră-fē)	process of recording spinal cord or bone marrow (activity)
neur/o	nerve	neurocytoma (nū-rō-sī-TŌ-mă)	tumor of nerve cells
spin/o	spine	spinal stenosis (SPĪ-năl stě-NŌ-sĭs)	pertaining to an abnormal condition of narrowing or stricture of the spinal cord

STOP HERE.
Select the Combining Form Flash Cards for Chapter 3, and run through them at least 3 times before you continue.

PRACTICE EXERCISES

Use Table 3-1 to fill in the answers below.

1. _____ a tumor of the meninges

2. _____ gluelike tumor

3. _____ pertaining to the brain and vessels

4. _____ inflammation of the meninges

5. _____ process of recording spinal cord activity

6. _____ tumor of nerve cells

7. _____ herniation of the brain

8. _____ pertaining to an abnormal condition of narrowing or stricture of the spinal cord

9. Fill in the blanks with the appropriate anatomical terms and/or combining form.

A. Brain

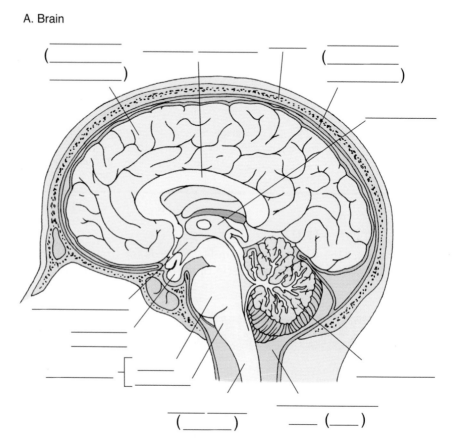

Figure 3-3

B. Spinal cord

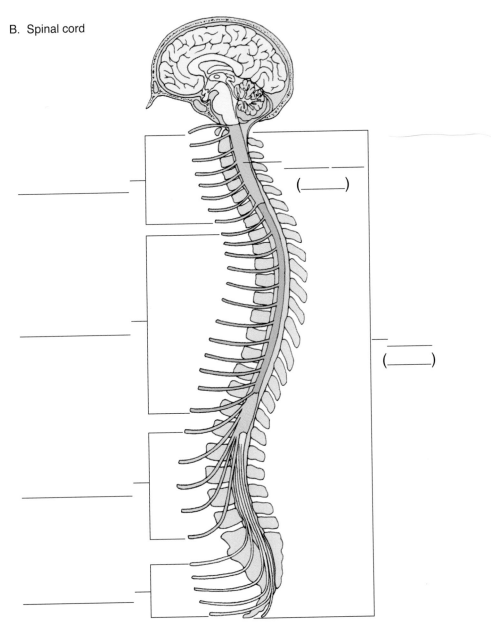

Figure 3-3 (Continued)

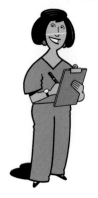

10. Fill in the blanks with the appropriate anatomical term.

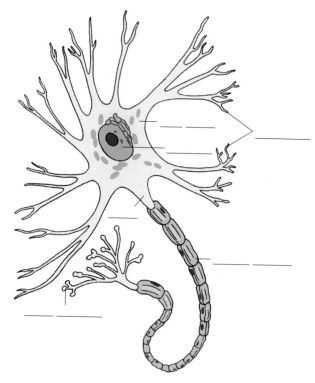

Figure 3-4

ABBREVIATIONS

Table 3-2 lists some of the most common abbreviations related to the nervous system as well as others often used in medical documentation.

TABLE 3-2	
ABBREVIATIONS	
ALS	amyotrophic lateral sclerosis (Lou Gehrig's disease)
CNS	central nervous system
CSF	cerebrospinal fluid
CT	computed tomography
CVA	cerebrovascular accident

EEG	electroencephalography
EMG	electromyogram
LP	lumbar puncture
MRI	magnetic resonance imaging
MS	multiple sclerosis
PNS	peripheral nervous system

STOP HERE.
Select the Abbreviation Flash Cards for Chapter 3, and run through them at least 3 times before you continue.

PATHOLOGY TERMS

Table 3-3 lists terms that relate to diseases or abnormalities of the nervous system. Use the pronunciation guide, and say the terms out loud as you read them. This will help you get in the habit of saying them properly.

TABLE 3-3
PATHOLOGY TERMS

Alzheimer's disease (ĂLTS-hī-mĕrz)	a form of chronic, progressive dementia caused by atrophy of brain tissue
Bell's palsy (PAWL-zē)	a form of facial paralysis, usually unilateral and temporary (Fig. 3-5)

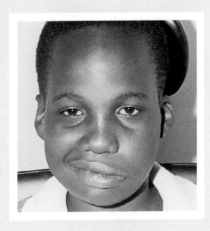

Figure 3-5 Bell's palsy. (From Dillon PM: Nursing Health Assessment. Philadelphia, FA Davis, p 218. Courtesy of Wills Eye Hospital.)

(text continues on page 58)

cerebrovascular (sĕr-ĕ-brō-VĂS-kū-lăr) **accident (CVA)**	damage or death of brain tissue caused by interruption of blood supply due to a clot or vessel rupture; also known as stroke or brain attack
epilepsy (ĔP-ĭ-lĕp-sē)	brain disorder characterized by recurrent seizures
Huntington's chorea (kō-RĒ-ă)	hereditary nervous disorder that leads to bizarre, involuntary movements and dementia
multiple sclerosis (MS) (sklĕ-RŌ-sĭs)	a disease involving progressive myelin degeneration, which results in loss of muscle strength and coordination
Parkinson's disease	progressive, degenerative disorder that results in tremors, gait changes and, occasionally, dementia
poliomyelitis (pōl-ē-ō-mī-ĕl-Ī-tĭs)	inflammation of the spinal cord by a virus, which may result in spinal and muscle deformity and paralysis
sciatica (sī-ĂT-ĭ-kă)	severe sciatic nerve pain that radiates from the buttocks to the feet (Fig. 3-6)

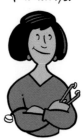

"Notice how the pain in sciatica radiates along the nerve pathways."

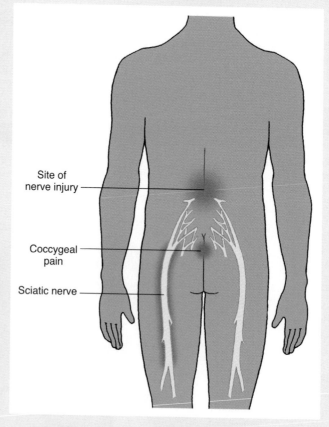

Figure 3-6 Radiation of sciatic nerve pain.

shingles (SHĬNG-lz)	unilateral painful vesicles, occurring on the upper body, caused by the herpes zoster virus (Fig. 3-7)

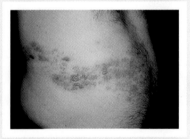

Figure 3-7 Herpes zoster. (From Goldsmith LA, Lazarus GS, Tharp MD: Adult and Pediatric Dermatology: A Color Guide to Diagnosis and Treatment. Philadelphia, FA Davis, 1997, p 307, with permission.)

spina bifida (SPĪ-nă BĪ-fĭd-ă)	incomplete closure of the spinal canal that may allow protrusion of the spinal cord and meninges at birth, leading to paralysis (Fig. 3-8)

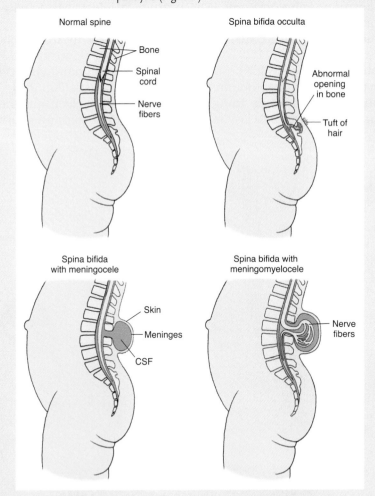

Normal spine

Bone

Spinal cord

Nerve fibers

Spina bifida occulta

Abnormal opening in bone

Tuft of hair

Spina bifida with meningocele

Skin

Meninges

CSF

Spina bifida with meningomyelocele

Nerve fibers

Figure 3-8 Spina bifida (neural tube defects).

transient ischemic (ĭs-KĒ-mĭk) attack (TIA)	temporary strokelike symptoms caused by a brief interruption of blood supply to a part of the brain

STOP HERE.
Select the Pathology Term Flash Cards for Chapter 3, and run through them at least 3 times before you continue.

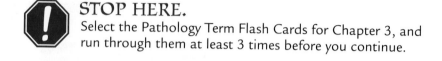

COMMON DIAGNOSTIC TESTS

Cerebrospinal fluid (CSF) analysis: analysis of fluid for blood, bacteria, and other abnormalities

Computed tomography (CT): study of the brain and spinal cord using radiology and computer analysis

Electroencephalography (EEG): study of electrical activity of the brain

Electromyogram (EMG): record of muscle activity from electrical stimulation

Lumbar puncture (LP): puncture of subarachnoid layer at 4th intervertebral space to obtain CSF fluid for analysis (Fig. 3-9)

Magnetic resonance imaging (MRI): uses an electromagnetic field and radio waves to create visual images on a computer screen

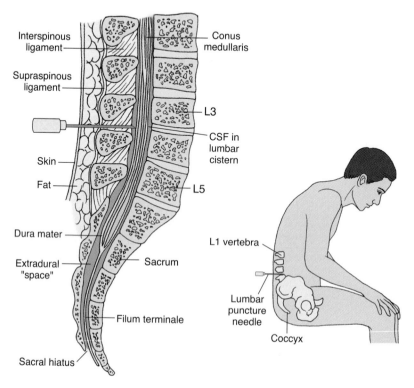

Figure 3-9 Lumbar puncture.

CASE STUDY

Read the following case study, and answer the questions that follow. Most of the terms are included in this chapter. Refer to the Glossary or to your medical dictionary for the other terms.

Shingles

Nicole Daniels is an 18-year-old female who developed a rash several days ago. She described it as a narrow strip of "tiny bumps" on the right side of her chest. Initially she noticed pruritis. Today she presented with a strip of herpetic vesicles that she describes as "exquisitely painful" with a sensation like a "fiery itch." She complained of sensitivity so severe that wearing clothing was painful because she could barely tolerate anything touching her skin. After completing a Hx and PE, her physician diagnosed her with shingles. He prescribed acyclovir to reduce the viral shedding and neuralgia. He also gave Nicole a prescription for acetaminophen with codeine to help relieve her pain.

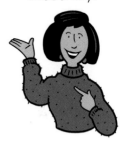

"Oh, good, another case study!"

Shingles is caused by the reactivation of the varicella virus years after an initial outbreak of chickenpox. A painful eruption of vesicles occurs along the course of a segment of a spinal or cranial peripheral nerve. The lesions are nearly always unilateral. The trunk is most often affected, but the face and head may also be involved. After an outbreak of chickenpox, the virus lies dormant in the nerve cells. Individuals with a weakened immune system (from AIDS, cancer, etc.) are more vulnerable to outbreaks. Pain may continue for months after the lesions heal. This is known as postherpetic neuralgia. Fortunately, recurrent outbreaks of shingles are rare.

Case Study Questions

1. What did Nicole first notice on the side of her chest?
   a. Papules
   b. Scales
   c. Macules
   d. Vesicles

2. After a few days, the "tiny bumps" turned into
   a. Scales
   b. Bigger bumps
   c. Blisters
   d. Scabs

3. Nicole has neuralgia, which is
   a. Itching
   b. Nerve pain
   c. Fatigue
   d. Nerve paralysis

(continues on page 60)

4. Chickenpox is caused by
   a. The varicella virus
   b. A bacterial infection from chickens
   c. AIDS
   d. A fungus

5. The pattern of the outbreak is usually unilateral. This means that it is
   a. On both sides of the body
   b. On one side of the body
   c. All over the body
   d. On the upper half of the body

6. People who are most vulnerable to shingles outbreaks are those
   a. With strong immune systems
   b. With weakened immune systems
   c. Who have had rubella
   d. Who have had measles

7. Recurrences of shingles outbreaks are common.   True   False

WEB SITES

National Spinal Cord Injury Association: www.spinalcord.org
National Parkinson Foundation: www.parkinson.org
National Multiple Sclerosis Society: www.nmss.org
Brain Trauma Foundation: www.aneuroa.org
Alzheimer's Association: www.alz.org

PREFIX AND SUFFIX REVIEW

Tables 3-4 and 3-5 contain a review of selected prefixes and suffixes. Refer to these tables as you complete the practice exercises at the end of the chapter.

TABLE 3-4
PREFIX PRONUNCIATIONS AND MEANINGS

Prefix	Pronunciation Guide	Meaning
a-, an-, in-	ā, ăn, ĭn	without, absence of
dys-	dĭs	painful, difficult
eu-	ū	good, normal
hemi-	hĕm-ē	half
infra-	ĭn-fră	positioned beneath
iso-	ī-sō	same, equal
poly-	pŏl-ē	many, much
para-	păr-ă	near, surrounding
quadri-	kwŏd-rĭ	four

TABLE 3-5
SUFFIX PRONUNCIATIONS AND MEANINGS

Suffix	Pronunciation Guide	Meaning
-al, -ic, -ous	ăl, ĭk, ŭs	pertaining to
-algia	ăl-jē-ă	pain
-cele	sēl	hernia
-cyte	sīt	cell
-graphy	gră-fē	process of recording
-itis	ī-tĭs	inflammation
-oma	ō-mă	tumor
-osis	ō-sĭs	abnormal condition
-paresis	păr-ē-sĭs	slight or partial paralysis
-pathy	pă-thē	disease
-phagia	fā-jē-ă	eating, swallowing
-phasia	fā-zē-ă	speech
-plegia	plē-jē-ă	paralysis

PRACTICE EXERCISES

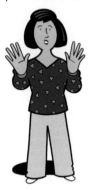

"To get the most out of these exercises, be sure to check your answers only AFTER you are done."

Complete the following practice exercises. The answers can be found in Appendix G.

Matching

Match the following combining forms with the correct meanings. Some answers may be used more than once or not at all.

1. _____ gli/o   a. brain

2. _____ myel/o   b. nerve

3. _____ mening/o   c. vertebra

4. _____ encephal/o   d. spine

5. _____ cerebr/o   e. spinal cord, bone marrow

6. _____ neur/o   f. meninges

7. _____ spin/o   g. glue or gluelike

Word Building

*Using **only** the word parts in the lists provided, create medical terms with the indicated meanings.*

Prefixes	**Combining Forms**	**Suffixes**
quadri-	electr/o	-al
hemi-	encephal/o	-algia
infra-	gli/o	-cele
iso-	mening/o	-ic
para-	myel/o	-itis
poly-	neur/o	-oma
	spin/o	-ous
		-paresis
		-pathy
		-plegia

1. much nerve inflammation _____

2. pertaining to positioned beneath the
   spine _____

3. herniation of the spinal cord and
   meninges _____

4. inflammation of the brain and
   meninges _____

5. pertaining to near the spine _____

6. tumor of nerve glue _____

7. pertaining to the same electric _____

8. half (body) partial paralysis _____

9. paralysis of four extremities _____

10. paralysis of two extremities _____

11. disease of the brain _____

12. nerve pain _____

Deciphering Terms

Write the correct translation of the following medical terms.

1. cerebrospinal _____

2. neuropathy _____

3. myeloma _____

4. meningitis _____

5. encephalography _____

6. gliocyte _____

7. cerebrosclerosis _____

8. hemiplegia _____

9. paraplegic _____

10. quadriparesis _____

11. neuritis _____

True or False

Decide whether the following statements are true or false.

1. True   False   **CT** stands for crainothoracic.

2. True   False   **CNS** stands for central nervous system.

3. True   False   **Epilepsy** is a brain disorder characterized by recurrent seizures.

4. True   False   A form of facial paralysis affecting one or both sides of the face, which is usually temporary, is known as **Bell's palsy.**

5. True   False   A **transient ischemic attack (TIA)** causes death of affected brain cells.

6. True   False   A **shingles** outbreak is caused by the herpes zoster virus.

7. True   False   A **CVA** results in death of affected brain cells.

8. True   False   **Sciatica** causes nerve pain in the buttocks and legs.

9. True   False   **Spina bifida** may cause paralysis.

10. True   False   **Huntington's chorea** causes inflammation of the spinal cord by a virus that may result in spinal and muscle deformity and paralysis.

Fill in the Blank

Fill in the blanks below.

1. A term that means *seizure disorder* is _____.

2. A temporary form of facial paralysis that is usually unilateral is _____.

3. A(n) _____ results in the death of brain cells.

4. Incomplete closure of the spinal canal is known as

   _____.

5. A(n) _____ causes mild, temporary strokelike symptoms.

6. _____ is a hereditary nervous disorder that results in bizarre involuntary movements and dementia.

Common Diagnostic Tests

Write the definition of the following diagnostic tests.

"You're doing great! Keep going!"

1. **Cerebrospinal fluid (CSF) analysis:**

2. **Computed tomography (CT):**

3. **Electroencephalography (EEG):**

4. **Electromyogram (EMG):**

5. **Lumbar puncture (LP):**

6. **Magnetic resonance imaging (MRI):**

Multiple Choice Questions

Select the best answer to the following multiple choice questions.

1. Mrs. Fritz was hospitalized with a CVA. She is currently comatose and unresponsive. To determine whether she still has meaningful brain activity, the physician will most likely order a(n)

   a. EMG

   b. LP

   c. CFS

   d. EEG

2. Ms. Yee sustained a CVA to the left side of her brain. Because of this, she currently has diminished sensation and movement on her right side. The proper term for this is

   a. Left hemiparalysis

   b. Left hemiparesis

   c. Right hemiparesis

   d. Right hemiparalysis

3. Mr. Stutzman is recovering from a CVA but still has difficulty speaking. The proper term for this is

   a. Dysphasia

   b. Dysphagia

   c. Aphasia

   d. Aphagia

4. Mrs. Villanueva is recovering from a CVA but is still struggles with swallowing. The proper term for this is

   a. Dysphasia

   b. Dysphoria

   c. Euphagia

   d. Dysphagia

5. Mr. Washington was brought to the emergency department with a high fever, confusion, and a headache. The physician wants to obtain a specimen of cerebrospinal fluid to study it for the presence of blood, bacteria, or other abnormalities. What procedure is the physician most likely to perform?

a. MRI

b. LP

c. EMG

d. CT

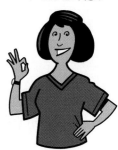

"You've completed the whole chapter. You're a real winner!"

4 CARDIOVASCULAR AND LYMPHATIC SYSTEMS

STRUCTURE AND FUNCTION OF THE CARDIOVASCULAR SYSTEM

The key function of the heart is to pump blood that is rich in oxygen and nutrients to the trillions of cells of the human body. To accomplish this, the heart beats an average of 60 to 90 times a minute for your entire lifetime. The heart is a very muscular organ with four chambers (Fig. 4-1). The **atria** are the two upper chambers that do approximately 30% of the workload. They contract with each heartbeat, pumping blood into the two lower chambers, which are called the **ventricles.** The ventricles have thicker, more muscular walls because they accomplish the other 70% of the workload. The right ventricle **(RV)** pumps blood that has returned from the body to the lungs, where it gets rid of carbon dioxide **(CO_2)** and picks up oxygen **(O_2).** The left ventricle **(LV)** pumps the oxygen-rich blood, fresh from the lungs, out to the various parts of the body. The walls of the left ventricle have even thicker walls than the right ventricle because it must work harder to pump blood further.

As oxygen-rich blood is pumped from the heart, it travels to all parts of the body through an intricate network of arteries. The arteries vary in size, from the very large aorta to very tiny arterioles. From the arterioles, the blood enters numerous microscopic-sized capillary beds with walls that are just one cell thick. This allows oxygen and nutrients to leave the capillaries and enter the tissues and cells and allows waste products and CO_2 to cross from the cells and tissues back into the capillaries. Blood that is now low in O_2 and high in CO_2 and waste leaves the capillaries and enters microscopic-sized venules (tiny veins). As it continues on its return journey, the blood travels through larger and larger veins

"The left ventricle does most of the work."

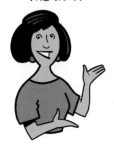

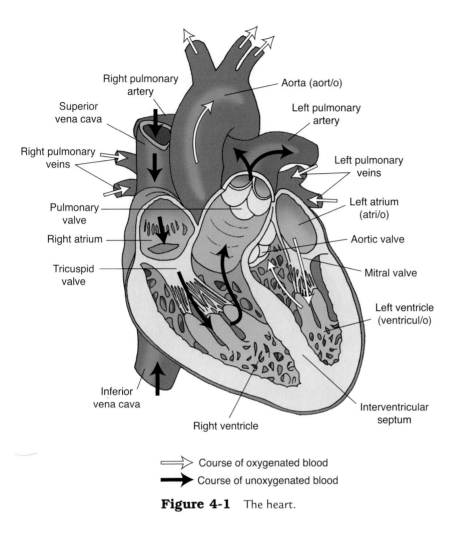

Right pulmonary artery

Aorta (aort/o)

Superior vena cava

Left pulmonary artery

Right pulmonary veins

Left pulmonary veins

Pulmonary valve

Left atrium (atri/o)

Right atrium

Aortic valve

Tricuspid valve

Mitral valve

Left ventricle (ventricul/o)

Inferior vena cava

Interventricular septum

Right ventricle

⇒ Course of oxygenated blood
⟹ Course of unoxygenated blood

Figure 4-1 The heart.

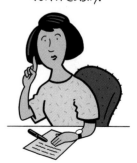

"The walls of the capillaries are extremely thin, which allows gases, nutrients, and wastes to cross back and forth easily."

until it reaches the heart. Blood is drained from the head and upper body via the superior vena cava and from the lower body via the inferior vena cava (Fig. 4-2).

The heart is surrounded by a fibrous membrane known as the pericardium or pericardial sac, which contains a very small amount of pericardial fluid. Occasionally, inflammation may develop within the pericardial sac. This condition is called **pericarditis.**

The heart has its own network of coronary vessels that keep it supplied with oxygen and nutrients. Occasionally, **arteriosclerosis** develops in these vessels, and they become narrowed and hardened due to a number of factors, including **hypertension**

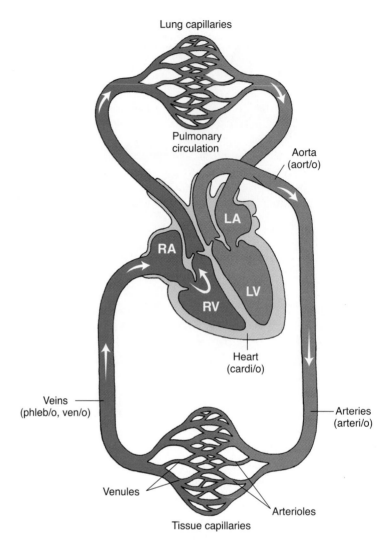

Figure 4-2   The cardiovascular system.

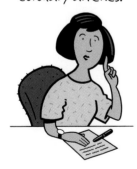

"The heart has its own special source of blood, oxygen, and nutrients: the coronary arteries."

(high blood pressure). In addition, a fatty plaquelike substance composed of **cholesterol** may build up on the inside surfaces of coronary vessels, causing further narrowing or even blockage. This is known as **atherosclerosis** and contributes to the development of **coronary artery disease (CAD).** It is also sometimes called atherosclerotic heart disease **(ASHD).** If a vessel becomes completely **occluded** (blocked), then the heart muscle downstream dies from lack of oxygen. This is known as a **myocardial infarction (MI)** or a heart attack.

STRUCTURE AND FUNCTION OF THE LYMPHATIC SYSTEM

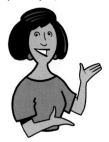

"The lymph nodes (glands) work like little filters, cleaning foreign matter from your lymph fluid."

The lymphatic system includes an intricate network of lymph vessels that collect excess tissue fluid and return it to circulation. It also plays a major role in the immune system as it cleanses the fluid called **lymph.** There are numerous **lymph nodes,** commonly called **glands,** distributed along the lymph system (Fig. 4-3). These nodes act as filters because they are rich in **white blood cells (WBCs),** which literally gobble up or engulf the bacteria and

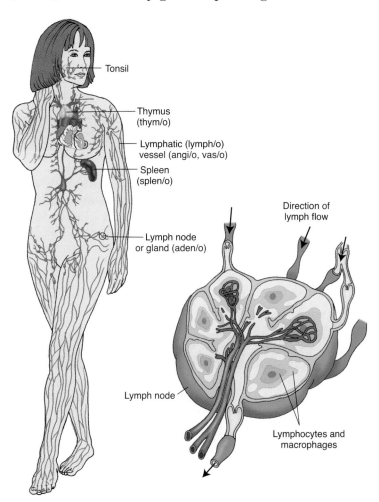

Tonsil

Thymus (thym/o)

Lymphatic (lymph/o) vessel (angi/o, vas/o)

Spleen (splen/o)

Lymph node or gland (aden/o)

Direction of lymph flow

Lymph node

Lymphocytes and macrophages

Figure 4-3   The lymphatic system.

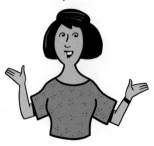

"Most people can get along fine without the spleen."

cellular debris through a process called **phagocytosis.** There are two sets of lymph nodes in the oropharynx. These are commonly known as the **tonsils** and **adenoids.** You may have noticed that these nodes occasionally become tender and swollen when you have a cold or sore throat. This is because they have been hard at work filtering bacteria, viruses, or other substances from your lymph fluid. Occasionally, they are overwhelmed and become inflamed and tender as a result.

Other structures involved in the lymphatic system include the **thymus** and the **spleen.** The thymus is most active when we are young, and it plays a role in cellular immunity. The spleen is a useful, yet expendable, organ that contains a ready supply of extra **red blood cells (RBCs)** and WBCs. Because of its location and rich blood supply, the spleen is sometimes injured when a person sustains a blow to the abdomen. Such an injury may require a splenectomy to stop the internal bleeding. Fortunately, we can usually get along quite nicely without a spleen.

COMBINING FORMS

Table 4-1 contains combining forms that pertain to the cardiovascular and lymphatic systems, examples of terms that utilize the combining form, and a pronunciation guide. Read out loud to yourself as you move from left to right across the table. Be sure to use the pronunciation guide so that you can learn to say the terms correctly.

TABLE 4-1

COMBINING FORMS CARDIOVASCULAR/ LYMPHATIC SYSTEM

Combining Form	Meaning	Example (Pronunciation)	Meaning of New Term
aden/o	gland	adenoma (ăd-ĕ-NŌ-mă)	tumor of a gland
angi/o	vessel	angioedema (ăn-jē-ō-ĕ-DĒ-mă)	swelling of a vessel
vas/o		vasorrhaphy (văs-OR-ă-fē)	suture of a vessel

Combining Form	Meaning	Example (Pronunciation)	Meaning of New Term
aort/o	aorta	aortostenosis (ā-or-tō-stĕ-NŌ-sĭs)	narrowing or stricture of the aorta
arteri/o	artery	arteriosclerosis (ăr-tē-rē-ō-sklĕ-RŌ-sĭs)	abnormal condition of hardening of the artery
ather/o	thick, fatty	atheroma (ăth-ĕr-Ō-mă)	thick, fatty tumor
atri/o	atria	atrioventricular (ā-trē-ō-vĕn-TRĬK-ū-lăr)	pertaining to the atria and the ventricles
cardi/o	heart	tachycardia (tăk-ē-KĂR-dē-ă)	a condition of a rapid heart (beat)
electr/o	electric	electrocardiogram (ē-lĕk-trō-KĂR-dē-ō-grăm)	record of electric (activity of the) heart
hem/o	blood	hemolytic (hē-mō-LĬT-ĭk)	pertaining to destruction of the blood
hemat/o		hematemesis (hĕm-ăt-ĔM-ĕ-sĭs)	vomiting of blood
lymph/o	lymph	lymphoma (lĭm-FŌ-mă)	lymph tumor
phleb/o	vein	phleborrhexis (flĕb-ō-RĔK-sĭs)	rupture of the vein
ven/o		venostasis (vē-nō-STĀ-sĭs)	stopping of a vein (refers to slowed blood flow)
splen/o	spleen	splenomegaly (splē-nō-mē-GĂ-lē)	enlargement of the spleen
thromb/o	thrombus (clot)	thrombophlebitis (thrŏm-bō-flē-BĪ-tĭs)	inflammation of a vein with presence of a clot
ventricul/o	ventricle	ventriculostomy (vĕn-trĭk-ū-LŎS-tō-mē)	mouthlike opening in the ventricle

STOP HERE.
Select the Combining Form Flash Cards for Chapter 4, and run through them at least 3 times before you continue.

"Ok, time to practice. Ready? Go!"

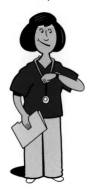

PRACTICE EXERCISES

Use Table 4-1 to fill in the answers below.

1. _____ mouthlike opening in the ventricle

2. _____ swelling of a vessel

3. _____ a condition of a rapid heart (beat)

4. _____ enlargement of the spleen

5. _____ record of electric (activity of the) heart

6. _____ abnormal condition of hardening of the artery

7. _____ rupture of the vein

8. _____ suture of a vessel

9. _____ thick fatty tumor

10. _____ vomiting of blood

11. _____ tumor of a gland

12. _____ lymph tumor

13. _____ narrowing or stricture of the aorta

14. _____ stopping of a vein (refers to slowed blood flow)

15. _____ pertaining to the atria and the ventricles

16. _____ pertaining to destruction of the blood

17. _____ inflammation of a vein with presence of a clot

18. Fill in the blanks with the appropriate anatomical term and/or combining form (Fig. 4-4).

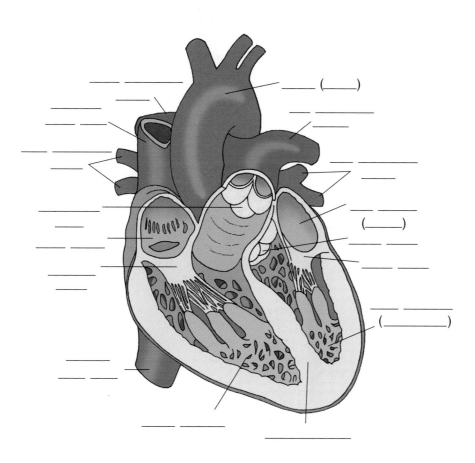

Figure 4-4

19. Fill in the blanks with the appropriate anatomical term and/or combining form (Fig. 4-5).

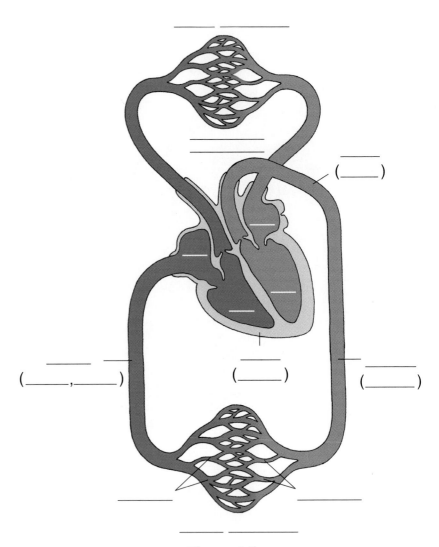

Figure 4-5

20. Fill in the blanks with the appropriate anatomical term and/or combining form (Fig. 4-6).

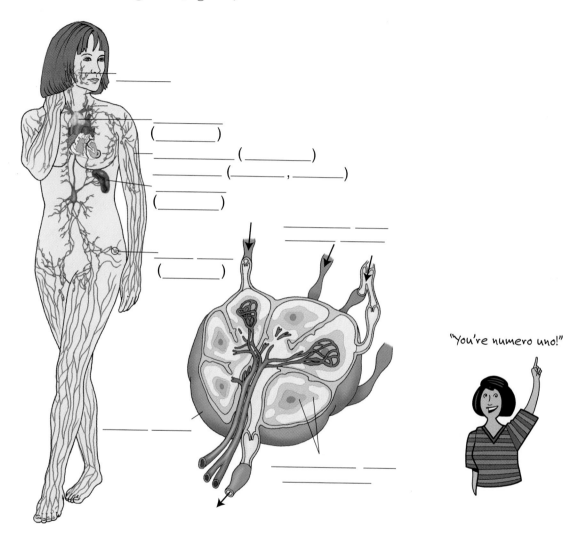

"You're numero uno!"

Figure 4-6

ABBREVIATIONS

Table 4-2 lists some of the most common abbreviations related to the cardiovascular and lymphatic systems as well as others often used in medical documentation.

TABLE 4-2
ABBREVIATIONS

Cardiovascular System

ASHD	arteriosclerotic heart disease
BP	blood pressure
CABG	coronary artery bypass graft (Fig. 4-7)

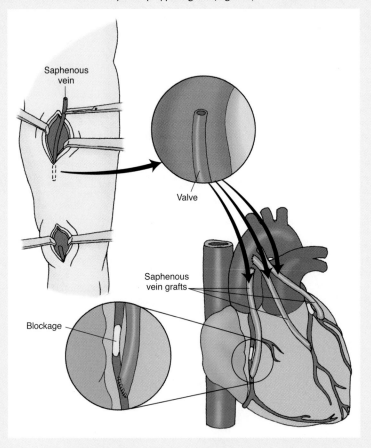

Figure 4-7   Coronary artery bypass graft.

CAD	coronary artery disease
CHF	congestive heart failure

ECG, EKG	electrocardiogram
HTN	hypertension (high blood pressure)
INR	international normalized ratio
LA	left atrium
LV	left ventricle
MI	myocardial infarction
PTCA	percutaneous transluminal coronary angioplasty (Fig. 4-8)

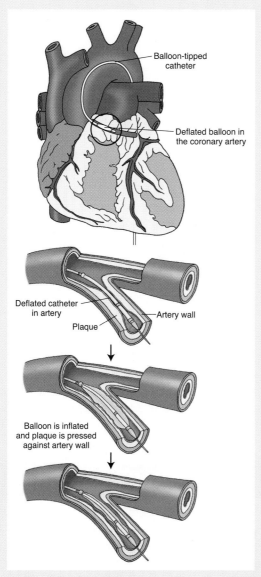

Figure 4-8 Percutaneous transluminal coronary angioplasty.

(continues on page 80)

ABBREVIATIONS *(Continued)*

Cardiovascular System

PT	prothrombin time
PTT	partial thromboplastin time
RA	right atrium
ROM	range of motion
RV	right ventricle

Lymphatic System

AIDS	acquired immunodeficiency syndrome
HIV	human immunodeficiency virus
PCP	*Pneumocystis carinii* pneumonia

Dosing Times

bid	twice a day
qid	four times a day
tid	three times a day
qh	every hour
q2h	every 2 hours
qhs	each evening (hour of sleep)
qam	each morning

"Be very careful with dosing abbreviations. Clarity here is critical."

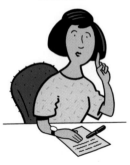

STOP HERE.
Select the Abbreviation Flash Cards for Chapter 4, and run through them at least 3 times before you continue.

PATHOLOGY TERMS

Table 4-3 includes terms that relate to diseases or abnormalities of the cardiovascular and lymphatic systems. Use the pronunciation guide, and say the terms out loud as you read them. This will help you get in the habit of saying them properly.

TABLE 4-3

PATHOLOGY TERMS

Cardiovascular System

aneurysm (ĂN-ū-rĭzm)	weakening and bulging of part of a vessel wall
arrhythmia (ă-RĬTH-mē-ă)	loss of heart rhythm (rhythm irregularity)
bruit (brwē)	soft blowing sound caused by turbulent blood flow in a vessel
congestive heart failure (CHF)	heart condition that results in lung congestion and dyspnea
deep vein thrombosis	development of a blood clot in a deep vein, usually in the legs
embolus (ĔM-bō-lŭs)	undissolved matter floating in blood or lymph fluid that may cause an occlusion and infarct
fibrillation (fĭ-brĭl-Ā-shŭn)	quivering of heart muscle fibers instead of an effective heart beat
hypertension (hī-pĕr-TĔN-shŭn)	blood pressure that is consistently higher than normal
ischemia (ĭs-KĒ-mē-ă)	temporary reduction in blood supply to a localized area of tissue
murmur (MŬR-mŭr)	blowing or swishing sound in the heart due to turbulent blood flow or backflow through a leaky valve
myocardial (mī-ō-KĂR-dē-ăl) **infarction**	death of heart muscle cells due to occlusion of a vessel (Fig. 4-9)

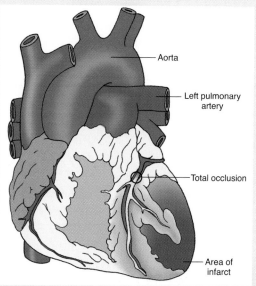

Aorta

Left pulmonary artery

Total occlusion

Area of infarct

Figure 4-9 Myocardial infarction.

(text continues on page 82)

Cardiovascular System

stroke (strōk)	death of brain cells due to loss of blood supply (also called brain attack)
transient ischemic (ĭs-KĒ-mĭk) **attack**	temporary strokelike symptoms caused by a brief interruption of blood supply to a part of the brain
varicose veins (VĂR-ĭ-kōs vāns)	bulging, distended veins due to incompetent valves, most commonly in the legs (Fig. 4-10)

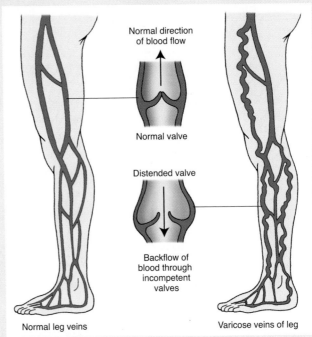

Normal direction of blood flow

Normal valve

Distended valve

Backflow of blood through incompetent valves

Normal leg veins

Varicose veins of leg

Figure 4-10   Varicose veins with incompetent valves.

Lymphatic System

acquired immunodeficiency syndrome	weakened state of the immune system, caused by human immunodeficiency virus
Hodgkin's disease	a type of lymphatic cancer
lymphosarcoma (lĭm-fō-săr-KŌ-mă)	cancer of lymphatic tissue not related to Hodgkin's disease
mononucleosis (mŏn-ō-nū-klē-Ō-sĭs)	acute infection of the Epstein-Barr virus, which causes sore throat, fever, fatigue, and enlarged lymph nodes

STOP HERE.
Select the Pathology Term Flash Cards for Chapter 4, and run through them at least 3 times before you continue.

COMMON DIAGNOSTIC TESTS

Cardiovascular System

Cardiac catheterization: evaluation of heart vessels and valves via the injection of dye that shows up under radiology (Fig. 4-11)

International normalized ratio (INR): standardized method of checking the prothrombin time (PT), a blood clotting factor that is used to monitor Coumadin therapy (Coumadin is a medication that slows clotting time)

Partial thromboplastin time (PTT): measures blood clotting time, used to monitor heparin therapy (heparin is another medication that slows clotting time)

Transesophageal echocardiography (TEE): a study of the heart via a probe placed in the esophagus

Troponin: most accurate blood test to confirm diagnosis of an MI

Lymphatic/Immune Systems

Enzyme-linked immunosorbent assay (ELISA): test for diagnosing HIV

Erythrocyte sedimentation rate (ESR): test that indicates inflammation in the body

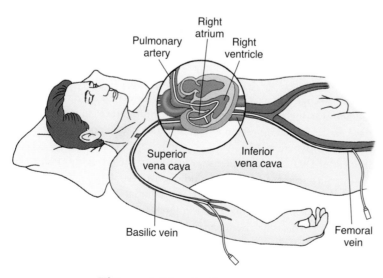

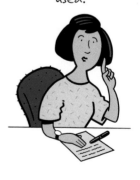

"For a cardiac cath, either the femoral or basilic vein may be used."

Figure 4-11 Cardiac catheterization.

CASE STUDY

Read the following case study, and answer the questions that follow. Most of the terms are included in this chapter. Refer to the Glossary or to your medical dictionary for the other terms.

Deep Vein Thrombosis

Arturo Espinoza is a 72-year-old retired cook with a history of ASHD and HTN. He also had an MI a year ago. He is 5' 9", weighs 220 lbs, and has been a pack-a-day smoker for 45 years. He recently noticed a deep, intense aching in his right lower leg but does not recall having injured it. Over the next few days, his right calf became tender and erythematous. In addition, his right lower leg, from the knee down, has become edematous.

After being evaluated by his family physician, Mr. Espinoza was diagnosed with a deep vein thrombosis (DVT) and started on SubQ heparin injection therapy bid. After several days of heparin therapy, Coumadin was started as well. Both PTT and INR levels were monitored. Once Mr. Espinoza achieved a therapeutic level on his Coumadin, he was able to discontinue the heparin. Coumadin therapy is planned for the next 3–6 months, and he will return on a monthly basis for monitoring.

Also known as **thrombophlebitis,** DVT occurs when a thrombus, or clot, develops in a vein and the vessel becomes inflamed. It can occur in any vein but is most common in the deep veins of the legs. Risk factors for a DVT include venous stasis from immobility, obesity, increased blood coagulability, and vascular injury. People with an increased risk include the elderly, smokers, and women over 30 years who use oral contraceptives.

Recently, increased attention has been paid to the occurrence of DVT among airline passengers. Some have called it *economy class syndrome* because of the prolonged sitting required of these passengers, which can cause venous stasis. This syndrome could be prevented if passengers were to be encouraged to exercise their feet and legs every 1-2 hours by walking in the aisles or doing range-of-motion exercises while sitting. Remaining well hydrated and wearing support hose are also helpful. (**Note:** support hose must have graduated compression and should **not** have a constricting band at the knee or anywhere else.)

Treatment of DVT may include rest, elevation of the extremity, and local heat application. Medications include nonsteroidal anti-inflammatory drugs (NSAIDs) and anticoagulant medication. Initial anticoagulant therapy includes heparin or Lovenox. Heparin levels must be monitored by checking the PTT. This is not necessary with Lovenox. After several days, warfarin (Coumadin) therapy is started. Blood levels of this medication are monitored by checking the INR. These medications slow the patient's blood-clotting time, which prevents further clot formation while the body's natural mechanisms dissolve the present clot. A potential side effect of these medications is easy bruising and increased risk of bleeding. Therefore, the patient must be counseled to watch for signs of bleeding; for example, on bowel movements or when brushing or flossing the teeth. If bleeding occurs, the physician should be notified.

Case Study Questions

1. What known risk factor for DVT does Mr. Espinoza have?
   a. He is a Mexican-American
   b. He is a smoker
   c. He is a man
   d. He is a retired cook

2. Mr. Espinoza has a history of what disorder?
   a. Atherosclerotic heart disease
   b. Diabetes
   c. Epilepsy
   d. *Pneumocystis carinii* pneumonia

3. By what route did Mr. Espinoza receive his heparin?
   a. By mouth
   b. Intramuscular injection
   c. Intradermal injection
   d. Subcutaneous injection

4. How often does Mr. Espinoza receive his heparin?
   a. Once each day
   b. Twice each day
   c. Three times each day
   d. Four times each day

5. What lab test was done to determine whether Mr. Espinoza's heparin dose was correct?
   a. PT
   b. PTT
   c. INR
   d. DVT

6. What lab test was done to determine whether Mr. Espinoza's Coumadin dose was correct?
   a. PT
   b. PTT
   c. INR
   d. DVT

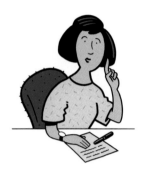

"How did you do on case?"

(continues on page 86)

7. Treatment of DVTs includes which of the following measures?
   a. Application of cold therapy
   b. Vigorous exercise
   c. Nonsteroidal anti-inflammatory medication
   d. Topical application of creams or ointments

8. Why has *economy class syndrome* become a recent popular name for DVT?
   a. Because flying in airplanes at high altitudes causes blood clot formation
   b. Because passengers who sit in economy class generally do not move about for the duration of the flight
   c. Because all airlines passengers are at high risk for blood clot formation
   d. Because DVT happens only to airline passengers

9. People can reduce their risk for DVT formation by doing which of the following?
   a. Drinking less fluid
   b. Sitting and resting their legs whenever possible
   c. Taking oral contraceptives
   d. Losing excess body weight

"How did you do on this case?"

WEB SITES

American Heart Association: www.americanheart.org
National Institute of Allergy and Infectious Diseases (NIAID): www.niaid.nih.gov
National HIV/AIDS Hotline: www.ashastd.org/nah

PREFIX AND SUFFIX REVIEW

Tables 4-4 and 4-5 contain a review of selected prefixes and suffixes. Refer to these tables as you complete the practice exercises at the end of the chapter.

TABLE 4-4

PREFIXES
PREFIX PRONUNCIATIONS AND MEANINGS

Prefix	Pronunciation Guide	Meaning
brady-	brăd-ē	slow
micro-	mī-krō	small
tachy-	tăk-ē	rapid

TABLE 4-5

SUFFIX PRONUNCIATIONS AND MEANINGS

Suffix	Pronunciation Guide	Meaning	Write in the term
-ia, -ic, -tic	ē-ă, ĭk, tĭk	pertaining to	
-algia -dynia	ăl-jē-ă dĭn-ē-ă	pain	
-cele	sēl	hernia	
-cyte	sīt	cell	
-gram	grăm	record	
-graphy	gră-fē	process of recording	
-ia, -ism	ē-ă, ĭzm	condition	
-itis	ī-tĭs	inflammation	
-logist	lō-jĭst	specialist in the study of	
-lysis	lĭ-sĭs	destruction of	
-malacia	mă-lā-sē-ă	softening	
-megaly	mĕg-ă-lē	enlargement	
-oid	oyd	resembling	
-ole, -ule	ōl, ūl	small	
-osis	ō-sĭs	abnormal condition	
-pathy	pă-thē	disease	
-plasty	plăs-tē	surgical repair	
-rrhexis	rĕk-sĭs	rupture	
-stasis	stă-sĭs	stopping	
-tomy	tō-mē	cutting into, incision	
-uria	ū-rē-ă	urine	

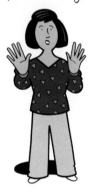

PRACTICE EXERCISES

Complete the following practice exercises. The answers can be found in Appendix G.

Matching

Match the following combining forms with the correct meanings. Some answers may be used more than once or not at all.

Exercise A

1. _____ arteri/o   a. gland

2. _____ ather/o   b. heart

3. _____ atri/o   c. vessel

4. _____ aort/o   d. atrium

5. _____ phleb/o   e. thick, fatty

6. _____ cardi/o   f. aorta

7. _____ angi/o   g. ventricle

8. _____ ven/o   h. artery

9. _____ aden/o   i. vein

Exercise B

1. _____ ventricul/o   a. spleen

2. _____ lymph/o   b. thrombus

3. _____ hemat/o   c. electric

4. _____ splen/o   d. vessel

5. _____ thromb/o   e. ventricle

6. _____ electr/o   f. vein

7. _____ hem/o   g. lymph

8. _____ angi/o   h. blood

Word Building

*Using **only** the word parts in the lists provided, create medical terms with the indicated meanings.*

Prefixes	**Combining Forms**	**Suffixes**
brady-	aden/o	-cele
tachy-	angi/o	-cyte
micro-	aort/o	-gram
	arteri/o	-graphy
	ather/o	-ia
	atri/o	-ic
	cardi/o	-logist
	electr/o	-megaly
	hemat/o	-oid
	lymph/o	-osis
	phleb/o	-pathy
	scler/o	-plasty
	splen/o	-rrhexis
	thromb/o	-sclerosis
	vas/o	-tomy
	ventricul/o	

1. record of a vessel _____

2. pertaining to the aorta _____

3. process of recording an artery _____

4. abnormal condition of hardening of thick, fatty
   (tissue) _____

5. rupture of the atrium _____

6. a condition of a slow heart (beat) _____

7. enlarged heart _____

8. a condition of a rapid heart (beat) _____

9. a record of heart electricity _____

10. specialist in the study of blood _____

11. resembling lymph _____

12. cutting into a vein _____

13. enlarged spleen _____

14. cell for clotting _____

15. surgical repair of a vessel _____

16. hernia of a ventricle _____

17. a disease of the glands _____

18. condition of a small heart _____

Deciphering Terms

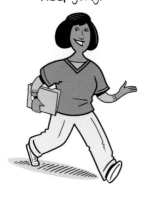

"You're doing great!
keep going!"

Write the correct translation of the following medical terms.

1. microcardia _____

2. venule _____

3. hemogram _____

4. angiography _____

5. aortoplasty _____

6. arteriole _____

7. atherocyte _____

8. atriodynia _____

9. electric _____

10. hematuria _____

11. lymphadenopathy _____

12. phlebitis _____

13. venostasis _____

14. splenomalacia _____

15. thrombolysis _____

16. vasalgia _____

17. ventriculoplasty _____

True or False

Decide whether the following statements are true or false.

1. True   False   The abbreviation **PTT** stands for platelets.

2. True   False   **Lymphosarcoma** is a type of cancer of lymphatic tissue not related to Hodgkin's disease.

3. True   False   A **murmur** is an abnormal blowing or swishing sound in the heart caused by turbulent blood flow or backflow through a leaky valve.

4. True   False   An **aneurysm** is a weakened area in the wall of a vessel.

5. True   False   The abbreviation **MI** stands for muscle injury.

6. True   False   The abbreviation **PTCA** stands for a type of food.

7. True False The abbreviation **CABG** stands for coronary artery bypass graft.

8. True False An **embolus** is a soft blowing sound caused by turbulent blood flow.

9. True False The abbreviation **CV** stands for coronary vessel.

10. True False **Ischemia** refers to a temporary reduction in blood supply to a localized area of tissue.

11. True False The abbreviation **ASHD** stands for arteriosclerotic heart disease.

12. True False **Fibrillation** refers to an abnormal quivering of heart muscle fibers instead of an effective heartbeat.

Fill in the Blank

Fill in the blanks below.

1. Jim's heart no longer beats in a regular rhythm. Therefore, he has a(n) _____.

2. A(n) _____ _____ _____, abbreviated _____, causes temporary strokelike symptoms due to temporary interference in blood supply to brain cells.

3. When the physician listened to Martha's carotid arteries with a stethoscope, he heard a *soft blowing sound caused by turbulent blood flow.* This is also known as a(n) _____.

4. The abbreviation *tid* stands for _____ _____ _____ _____.

5. Ismael has a *heart condition that results in lung congestion and dyspnea.* The medical term for this condition is

   _____ _____ _____.

6. The abbreviation *qhs* stands for _____ _____.

7. Victor was treated with an anticoagulant medication called heparin because of a *blood clot in a deep vein of his legs.* This condition is known as a(n) _____ _____ _____ and is abbreviated _____.

8. While Victor was taking heparin, a blood test was done regularly to check his *blood clotting time.* This test is known as the _____ _____ _____ and is abbreviated as _____.

"You learn by repetition, so keep going!"

9. The abbreviation *q2h* stands for _____ _____ _____.

10. The *death of heart muscle cells due to occlusion of a vessel* is known as a(n) _____ _____ and is abbreviated as _____.

11. Cristobalina has *bulging, distended veins* in her legs. This condition is known as _____

    _____.

12. *Hodgkin's disease* is a type of _____ _____.

13. The two upper chambers of the heart are abbreviated _____ and_____.

14. The two lower chambers of the heart are abbreviated _____ and _____.

15. Jaemoon has a history of *coronary artery disease*, which is abbreviated _____.

16. After checking Jaemoon's *BP* or _____ _____, the physician also diagnosed him with *HTN*, which stands for _____.

17. The physician ordered an *EKG* for Jaemoon. This stands for _____ and will record his heart rhythm.

18. A medication is ordered *qid*. This means it should be taken _____ times a day.

19. Oscar has become very ill with *AIDS*, which stands for _____ _____ _____.

20. Oscar got AIDS after becoming infected with the _____ _____ *virus*, which is abbreviated _____.

21. Oscar has developed a serious respiratory complication of AIDS, _____ _____ _____, which is abbreviated as *PCP*.

22. Treatment for PCP includes an antibiotic medication *bid*. This means that Oscar will take it _____ _____ _____.

23. The physician wants Oscar to weigh himself *qam*, which means _____ _____.

24. A(n) _____ causes death of brain cells due to loss of blood supply.

Common Diagnostic Tests

Write the definition of the following diagnostic tests.

Cardiovascular System

1. **Cardiac catheterization:**

2. **International normalized ratio (INR):**

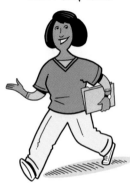

"You're almost done;
don't stop now."

3. **Partial thromboplastin time (PTT):**

4. **Transesopageal echocardiography (TEE):**

5. **Troponin:**

Lymphatic/Immune Systems

1. **Enzyme-linked immunosorbent assay (ELISA):**

2. **Erythrocyte sedimentation rate (ESR):**

Multiple Choice Questions

Select the best answer to the following multiple choice questions.

1. Which of the following disorders does **NOT** involve an interference of blood flow?

   a. Ischemia

   b. Myocardial infarction

   c. Stroke

   d. Arrhythmia

2. Which of the following is a type of cancer?

   a. Hodgkin's disease

   b. CHF

   c. DVT

   d. TIA

3. Which of the following abbreviations stands for a chamber of the heart?

   a. BP

   b. EKG

   c. RA

   d. PCP

4. Which of the following is responsible for causing acquired immunodeficiency syndrome?

   a. HIV

   b. RV

   c. CAD

   d. LV

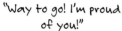

"Way to go! I'm proud of you!"

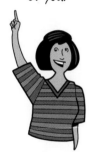

5. Which of the following may cause temporary strokelike symptoms?

   a. CHF

   b. TIA

   c. LA

   d. CPR

RESPIRATORY SYSTEM

5

STRUCTURE AND FUNCTION

Oxygen is essential for human life. Oxygen (O_2) is taken in through the act of breathing air into the lungs. Other terms for breathing in are *inspiration* and *inhalation*. Most of the time, breathing is an unconscious act. However, conscious control may be exerted, enabling us to take extra large breaths or even hold our breath for a short time. At some point, however, we have an overwhelming urge to breathe. This happens because when we stop breathing, carbon dioxide (CO_2) builds up in our blood. As this occurs, the pH level of the blood drops, reflecting increased acidity. To be our healthiest, our blood must remain slightly alkaline, within the narrow range of 7.35 to 7.45. As the pH level drops, we experience an urge to breathe. The act of inhalation brings fresh oxygen-rich air into the lungs so it can be absorbed into the blood.

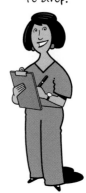

"Holding your breath causes the CO_2 level to rise and pH level to drop."

The act of breathing out, also known as *expiration* or *exhalation*, allows us to rid the body of the excess CO_2, thus restoring a normal blood pH level. Contrary to what most people think, the normal stimulus to breathe is not the lower oxygen levels in our blood, but the lowered pH level caused by CO_2 buildup.

Refer to Figure 5-1 as we discuss the path that air takes into and out of the body. The *upper airway* consists of the *mouth, nose, sinuses, nasopharynx,* and *oropharynx.* As air moves through these passages, it is warmed, filtered, and humidified. The air moves to the *lower airway* as it enters the *trachea.* From there it moves through the two primary *bronchi*, each of which leads to a lung. The bronchi split off into smaller bronchi and eventually into tiny *bronchioles.* The bronchioles end at the *alveoli,* which are microscopic-sized air sacs. There are approximately 300 million alveoli in each lung. They are covered with a delicate

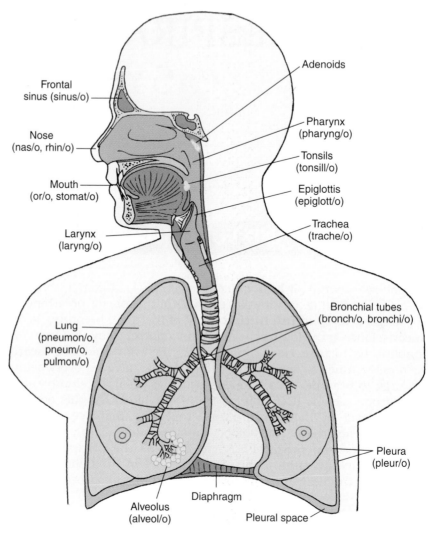

Figure 5-1   The respiratory system.

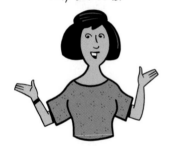

"Alveoli expand and contract similar to tiny balloons."

capillary bed (microscopic blood vessels) that provides a rich blood supply. The alveoli expand somewhat like tiny balloons during inspiration as air enters and fills them. They contract and partially deflate during expiration as much of the air moves out of the lungs. Because the walls of the alveoli and the capillary beds are each just one cell thick, gases move easily back and forth across them. Excess CO_2 leaves the capillaries and moves into the air space in the alveoli and is then exhaled. Oxygen moves from the air space in the alveoli into the capillary blood and is then distributed to various parts of the body via the circulatory system.

The two lungs are divided into lobes. The right lung has three lobes, and the left lung has two. Occasionally a person may be diagnosed with **lobar** pneumonia, which means that the pneumonia is confined to just one of these lobes. The lungs are covered with two thin membranes known as the **pleurae.** The **visceral pleura** lies directly on the lungs. The **parietal pleura** lines the inner wall of the thorax. Between the two membranes is a small amount of pleural fluid that helps the membranes slide smoothly against one another as the lungs expand and contract. The space between these two linings is sometimes referred to as a "potential" space because there is nothing there other than a small amount of this fluid. If there is an interruption in the integrity of one or both membranes, the person may develop a condition known to the layperson as a collapsed lung. The medical term for this condition is **pneumothorax,** if air has collected between the membranes, and **hemothorax,** if blood has collected there (Fig. 5-2).

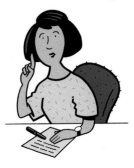

"A hole in the pleural membrane can cause air or fluid to collect, resulting in a collapsed lung."

COMBINING FORMS

Tables 5-1 and 5-2 contain combining forms that pertain to the respiratory system, examples of terms that utilize the combining form, and a pronunciation guide. Read out loud to yourself as you move from left to right across the table. Be sure to use the pronunciation guide so that you can learn to say the terms correctly.

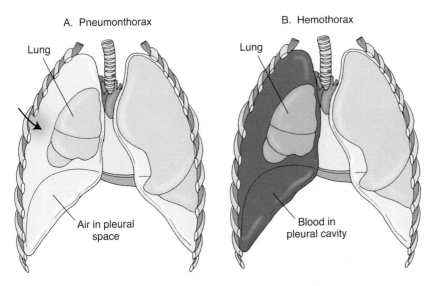

A. Pneumonthorax

Lung

Air in pleural space

B. Hemothorax

Lung

Blood in pleural cavity

Figure 5-2   *A, Pneumothorax. B, Hemothorax.*

TABLE 5-1

COMBINING FORMS RELATED TO THE RESPIRATORY SYSTEM

Combining Form	Meaning	Example	Meaning of New Term
bronch/o	bronchus	bronchitis (brŏng-KĪ-tĭs)	inflammation of the bronchus
bronchi/o		bronchiectasis (brŏng-kē-ĔK-tă-sĭs)	dilation or expansion of the bronchus
chondr/o	cartilage	chrondroplasty (KŎN-drō-plăs-tē)	surgical repair of the cartilage
epiglott/o	epiglottis	epiglottal (ĕp-ĭ-GLŎT-ăl)	pertaining to the epiglottis
laryng/o	larynx	laryngitis (lăr-ĭn-JĪ-tĭs)	inflammation of the larynx
nas/o	nose	nasogastric (nā-zō-GĂS-trĭk)	pertaining to the nose and stomach
rhin/o		rhinitis (rī-NĪ-tĭs)	inflammation of the nose (runny nose)
or/o	mouth	oral (Ō-răl)	pertaining to the mouth
stomat/o		stomatitis stō-mă-TĪ-tĭs	inflammation of the mouth
ox/o	oxygen	anoxia (ăn-ŎK-sē-ă)	condition of no oxygen
pharyng/o	pharynx	pharyngeal (făr-ĬN-jē-ăl)	pertaining to the pharynx
pleur/o	pleura	pleurodynia (ploo-rō-DĬN-ē-ă)	pain in the pleura
pneum/o	lung, air	pneumonia (nū-MŌ-nē-ă)	condition of the lung
pneumon/o		pneumonectomy (nū-mŏn-ĔK-tō-mē)	surgical excision of the lung
pulmon/o	lung	pulmonary (PŬL-mō-nĕ-rē)	pertaining to the lung
sinus/o	sinus	sinusoid (SĪ-nŭs-oyd)	resembling a sinus
thorac/o	thorax	thoracentesis (thō-ră-sĕn-TĒ-sĭs)	surgical puncture of the thorax
tonsill/o	tonsil	tonsillitis (tŏn-sĭl-Ī-tĭs)	inflammation of the tonsils
trache/o	trachea	tracheotomy (trā-kē-ŎT-ō-mē)	surgical incision into the trachea

TABLE 5-2			
OTHER COMBINING FORMS			
Combining Form	Meaning	Example	Meaning of New Term
aer/o	air	aerophagia (ĕr-ō-FĀ-jē-ă)	swallowing air
carcin/o	cancer	carcinoma (kăr-sĭ-NŌ-mă)	cancerous tumor
muc/o	mucus	mucoid (MŪ-koyd)	resembling mucus
orth/o	straight	orthopnea (or-THŎP-nē-ă)	breathing in the straight (upright) position

STOP HERE.

Select the Combining Form Flash Cards for Chapter 5, and run through them at least 3 times before you continue.

PRACTICE EXERCISES

Use Tables 5-1 and 5-2 to fill in the answers below.

1. _____ resembling mucus

2. _____ inflammation of the tonsils

3. _____ inflammation of the bronchus

4. _____ dilation or expansion of the bronchus

5. _____ pertaining to the epiglottis

6. _____ swallowing air

7. _____ pertaining to the pharynx

8. _____ surgical repair of the cartilage

9. _____ breathing in the straight (upright)
position

10. _____ pertaining to the nose and stomach

11. _____ cancerous tumor

12. _____ pertaining to the mouth

13. _____ condition of no oxygen

14. _____ condition of the lung

15. _____ inflammation of the nose (runny
nose)

16. _____ pain in the pleura

17. _____ pertaining to the lung

18. _____ resembling a sinus

19. _____ surgical puncture of the thorax

20. _____ surgical excision of the lung

21. _____ surgical incision into the trachea

22. _____ inflammation of the larynx

23. _____ inflammation of the mouth

24. Fill in the blanks with the appropriate anatomical terms and/or combining form.

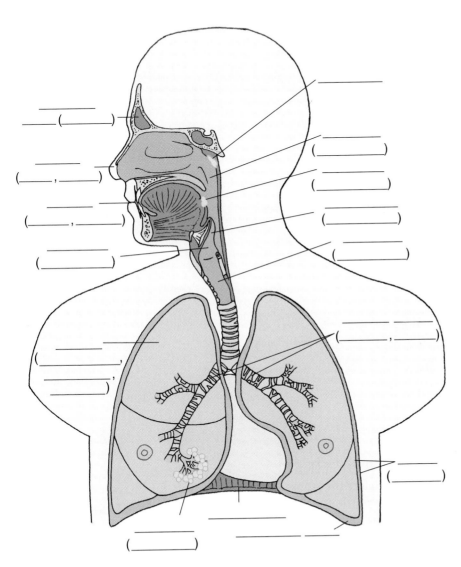

Figure 5-3

ABBREVIATIONS

Table 5-3 lists some of the most common abbreviations related to the respiratory system as well as others often used in medical documentation.

TABLE 5-3	
ABBREVIATIONS	
ABGs	arterial blood gases
ARDS	acute respiratory distress syndrome
COPD	chronic obstructive pulmonary disease
CPR	cardiopulmonary resuscitation
CO_2	carbon dioxide
O_2	oxygen
PND	paroxysmal nocturnal dyspnea
SARS	sudden acute respiratory syndrome
SOB	short of breath
stat	immediately
TB	tuberculosis
URI	upper respiratory infection
VC	vital capacity

"It's flash card time!"

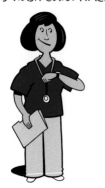

STOP HERE.
Select the Abbreviation Flash Cards for Chapter 5, and run through them at least 3 times before you continue.

PATHOLOGY TERMS

Table 5-4 includes terms that relate to diseases or abnormalities of the respiratory system. Use the pronunciation guide, and say the terms out loud as you read them. This will help you get in the habit of saying them properly.

TABLE 5-4

PATHOLOGY TERMS

acute respiratory distress syndrome	hypoxemia and respiratory failure due to severe inflammatory damage to the lungs; occurs after severe infection or trauma
sudden acute respiratory syndrome 🖉	viral respiratory illness marked by head and body aches, fever, and cough; may lead to severe pneumonia
asthma (ĂZ-mă)	disease marked by episodic narrowing and inflammation of the airways resulting in wheezing, SOB, and cough
chronic obstructive pulmonary disease	group of diseases in which alveolar air sacs are destroyed and chronic severe SOB results; smoking is a major cause (Fig. 5-4)

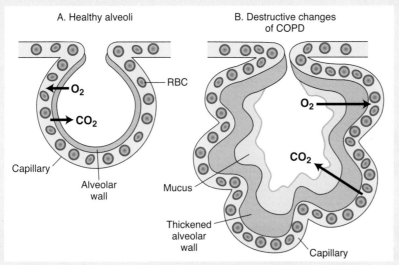

Figure 5-4 *A,* Normal alveoli. *B,* Destructive changes of COPD.

coryza (kŏ-RĪ-ză)	the common cold
crackles	abnormal crackly lung sound heard with a stethoscope; sounds like "rice krispies"
croup (croop)	an acute viral disease, usually in children, marked by a barking "seal-like" cough and respiratory distress
cystic fibrosis (SĬS-tĭk fī-BRŌ-sĭs)	fatal genetic disease that causes frequent respiratory infections, increased airway secretions, and COPD in children
empyema (ĕm-pī-Ē-mă)	collection of infected fluid (pus) in the pleural cavity
epistaxis (ĕp-ĭ-STĂK-sĭs)	a nosebleed

(continues on page 106)

PATHOLOGY TERMS *(Continued)*

hemothorax (hē-mō-THŌ-răks)	collection of blood or bloody fluid in the pleural cavity (see Fig. 5-2)
pleural effusion (PLOO-răl ĕ-FŪ-zhŭn)	collection of fluid in the pleural cavity
pneumothorax (nū-mō-THŌ-răks)	collection of air in the pleural cavity (see Fig. 5-2)
rhonchi (RŎNG-ī)	a coarse, gurgly sound heard in the lungs with a stethoscope, caused by secretions in the air passages
stridor (STRĪ-dor)	a high-pitched upper airway sound heard without a stethoscope; indicates airway obstruction—a medical emergency
wheeze (hwēz)	a somewhat musical sound heard in the lungs, usually with a stethoscope, caused by partial airway obstruction (such as with asthma)

STOP HERE.
Select the Pathology Term Flash Cards for Chapter 5, and run through them at least 3 times before you continue.

COMMON DIAGNOSTIC TESTS

Vital capacity (VC): measurement of volume of air that can be exhaled after maximum inspiration

Pulmonary angiography: radiographic examination of pulmonary circulation after injection of a contrast dye

Arterial blood gas (ABG): measures level of O_2, CO_2 and acid-base balance (pH) in arterial blood

Pulse oximetry: indirect measure of arterial blood O_2 saturation level, also known as the Spo_2; the normal level in a person with healthy lungs is 97% to 99%

Sputum analysis: examination of mucus or fluid coughed up from the lungs

CASE STUDY

Read the following case study, and answer the questions that follow. Most of the terms are included in this chapter. Refer to the Glossary or to your medical dictionary for the other terms.

Chronic Obstructive Pulmonary Disease (COPD)

Helga Freiderick is a 57-year-old woman who came to the urgent care clinic today complaining of SOB. On admission, her respirations were labored at a rate of 32. Her SpO_2 was just 84%, and her VC was decreased. She appeared anxious and stated that she "couldn't get enough air." Her lungs had bilateral expiratory wheezes throughout, scattered rhonchi, and bibasilar crackles. She had a frequent cough productive of thick green sputum.

Stat ABGs were drawn; she was put on O_2 at 2 lpm per NC and given a nebulizer Tx. A sputum specimen was collected and sent for C and S. She was given IV doses of a broad spectrum antibiotic and a steroid drug. Upon review of her ABGs, it was determined that she was in a state of mild respiratory acidosis.

A short time later, Mrs. Freidericks' respiratory rate had decreased to 20, her O_2 saturation was 91%, and she stated that she was breathing "much better." She was then transferred to the hospital for further monitoring and continued therapy.

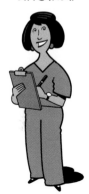

"You'll probably have many patients with COPD, so pay close attention."

COPD is a chronic disease with several different causes. The most common cause is smoking because the lungs are subjected to chronic irritation of an inhaled substance 20 to 40 times each day for years on end. As a result, the lung tissue becomes inflamed. Under normal circumstances, body tissue is able to repair itself. However, in the case of smoking, chronic, repeated exposure to the irritants prevents healing and results in chronic inflammation. Over time, permanent damage occurs. The walls of the delicate alveolae lose their elasticity and become permanently distended, like balloons that have been inflated too many times. The walls of the alveolae also erode and thicken and, as a result, function less effectively. They begin to trap air rather than allow it to escape during expiration. This decreases the amount of oxygen-rich air that can be inhaled in each breath.

As chronic air-trapping occurs, the chest changes dimension, becoming more barrel-like. The lungs also flatten on the bottom, robbing the diaphragm (an important respiratory muscle) of its effectiveness. Cilia in the airway normally move foreign debris upward to be coughed out. But in COPD, cilia become clogged with tar and lose effectiveness. As a result of these physical changes, the COPD patient may begin to experience some or all of the following symptoms:

(continues on page 108)

orthopnea: The need to remain upright in order to breathe effectively. Physicians often quantify the severity of orthopnea by referring to the number of pillows the patient must recline against while sleeping (3-pillow orthopnea).

hypercapnea: The chronic retention of CO_2. In some cases, this changes the way the person's body determines when to breathe. The person may begin to function according to the "hypoxic drive" and feel the urge to breathe when the O_2 level gets too low instead of when the CO_2 level gets too high. This becomes a problem when the person requires supplemental O_2. Too much O_2 can, in some circumstances, actually knock out the urge to breathe, leading to respiratory arrest. Furthermore, hypercapnea can lead to symptoms of mental cloudiness and lethargy.

chronic hypoxia: A chronic lack of oxygen. As gas exchange becomes less effective, breathing becomes more and more difficult. Eventually the person becomes dependent on oxygen. Yet, in the last stages of the disease, supplemental O_2 is of little help. The person feels chronically short of breath and becomes severely dyspneic with the slightest exertion.

Case Study Questions

1. Upon admission, Mrs. Freiderick was:
   a. Having chest pain
   b. Very short of breath
   c. Breathing very slowly
   d. Unconscious

2. Mrs. Freiderick had:
   a. An increased ability to breathe in
   b. A decreased ability to breathe in
   c. An increased ability to breathe out
   d. A decreased ability to breathe out

3. Mrs. Freidericks's oxygen saturation level was:
   a. Checked by pulse oximetry
   b. At a normal level
   c. Not known
   d. Higher than normal

4. When listening to Mrs. Freidericks's lungs, the physician heard:
   a. Normal sounds of air movement
   b. A somewhat musical sound caused by partial airway obstruction
   c. A high-pitched upper airway sound that indicates airway obstruction
   d. A barking "seal-like" cough

5. Which of the following statements is true?
   a. Mrs. Freiderick normally slept lying down
   b. It is always safe to give high levels of oxygen to people with COPD
   c. Supplemental O_2 effectively relieves dyspnea in the final stages of COPD
   d. Mrs. Freiderick's chest cavity had most likely become more barrel-like in shape

6. Which of the following statements is correct?
   a. Cilia continue to work effectively in people with late-stage COPD
   b. The only cause of COPD is smoking
   c. People with COPD tend to develop chronic O_2 retention
   d. Arterial blood was immediately drawn to analyze the levels of O_2, CO_2, and pH.

7. In a person with healthy lungs, the drive to breathe is stimulated by:
   a. Low levels of oxygen
   b. A drop in blood pH caused by high levels of CO_2
   c. A feeling of emptiness in the lungs
   d. A neurological message sent from the brain to the lungs

WEB SITES

Cystic Fibrosis Foundation: www.cff.org
American Lung Association: www.lungusa.org

PREFIX AND SUFFIX REVIEW

Tables 5-5 and 5-6 contain a review of selected prefixes and suffixes. Refer to these tables as necessary when you complete the exercises at the end of the chapter.

TABLE 5-5
PREFIX PRONUNCIATIONS AND MEANINGS

Prefix	Pronunciation Guide	Meaning
dys-	dĭs	painful, difficult
eu-	ū	good, normal
peri-	pĕr-ĭ	near, surrounding
tachy-	tăk-ē	rapid

TABLE 5-6
SUFFIX PRONUNCIATIONS AND MEANINGS

Suffix	Pronunciation Guide	Meaning
-al, -ary -ic, -tic -eal, -ous	ăl, ār-ē ĭk, tic ē-ăl, ŭs	pertaining to
-algia -dynia	ăl-jē-ă dĭn-ē-ă	pain
-centesis	sĕn-tē-sĭs	surgical puncture
-ectomy	ĕk-tō-mē	excision, surgical removal
-gen -genesis	jĕn jĕn-ĕ-sĭs	creating, producing
-ia, -ism	ē-ă, ĭzm	condition
-itis	ī-tĭs	inflammation
-lysis	lĭ-sĭs	destruction of
-malacia	mă-lā-sē-ă	softening
-oid	oyd	resembling
-oma	ō-mă	tumor
-osis	ō-sĭs	abnormal condition
-oxia	ŏk-sē-ă	oxygen
-pathy	pă-thē	disease
-pexy	pĕk-sē	surgical fixation
-phagia	fā-jē-ă	eating, swallowing
-phobia	fō-bē-ă	fear

Suffix	Pronunciation Guide	Meaning
-plegia	plē-jē-ă	paralysis
-pnea	pnē-ă	breathing
-scopy	skō-pē	visual examination
-stomy	stō-mē	mouthlike opening
-tome	tōm	cutting instrument
-tomy	tō-mē	cutting into, incision

PRACTICE EXERCISES

Complete the following practice exercises. The answers can be found in Appendix G.

"To get the most out of these exercises, be sure to check your answers only AFTER you are done."

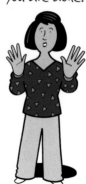

Matching

Match the following combining forms with the correct meanings. Some answers may be used more than once or not at all.

Exercise A

1. _____ bronch/o   a. nose

2. _____ or/o   b. mouth

3. _____ sinus/o   c. air

4. _____ chondr/o   d. cartilage

5. _____ epiglott/o   e. sinus

6. _____ rhin/o   f. cancer

7. _____ bronchi/o   g. straight

8. _____ aer/o   h. epiglottis

9. _____ nas/o   i. bronchus

Exercise B

1. _____ trache/o	a.	lung, air
2. _____ muc/o	b.	mucus
3. _____ carcin/o	c.	pleura
4. _____ tonsill/o	d.	thorax
5. _____ pleur/o	e.	larynx
6. _____ thorac/o	f.	trachea
7. _____ pharyng/o	g.	oxygen
8. _____ ox/o	h.	tonsil
9. _____ pneum/o	i.	pharynx
10. _____ laryng/o	j.	cancerous

Word Building

Using **only** the word parts in the lists provided, create medical terms with the indicated meanings.

Prefixes	**Combining Forms**	**Suffixes**
dys-	aer/o	-al
eu-	bronch/o	-ary
peri-	carcin/o	-dynia
tachy-	chondr/o	-gen
	cutane/o	-genesis
	epiglott/o	-ic
	laryng/o	-itis
	muc/o	-malacia
	myc/o	-oid
	nas/o	-oma
	pharyng/o	-osis
	pleur/o	-ous
	pneum/o	-pathy
	pulmon/o	-pexy
	sinus/o	-pnea
	thorac/o	-scopy
	tonsill/o	-stomy
	trache/o	-tomy

1. pertaining to the bronchus and lung _____

2. tumor of cartilage _____

3. creating air _____

4. pertaining to mucus and skin _____

5. visual examination of the trachea and
   bronchus _____

6. disease of the tonsils _____

7. softening of the trachea _____

8. inflammation of the epiglottis _____

9. pertaining to near the nose _____

10. pertaining to painful or difficult
    breathing _____

11. normal breathing _____

12. incision into the thorax _____

13. abnormal condition of throat fungus _____

14. painful pleurae _____

15. surgical fixation of the lungs _____

16. pertaining to the lungs _____

17. resembling the sinus _____

18. mouthlike opening in the trachea _____

19. pertaining to causing cancer _____

20. rapid breathing _____

21. visual examination of the larynx _____

"Muy bueno! You're
off to a sensational
start."

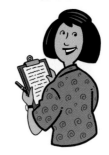

Deciphering Terms

Write the correct translation of the following medical terms.

1. laryngeal _____

2. pleuralgia _____

3. pneumatic _____

4. pneumonia _____

5. pulmonary _____

6. sinusotomy _____

7. thoracentesis _____

8. tonsillectomy _____

9. dyspnea _____

10. hemothorax _____

11. pneumothorax _____

12. eupnea _____

13. orthopnea _____

14. rhinitis _____

15. tracheostomy _____

16. aerophagia _____

17. pharyngeal _____

18. nasal _____

19. mucolysis _____

20. carcinoma _____

True or False

Decide whether the following statements are true or false.

1. True   False   The abbreviation **TB** stands for terminal bronchitis.

2. True   False   A **wheeze** is a musical sound in the lungs caused by an airway narrowing.

3. True   False   The abbreviation **SARS** stands for sudden acute respiratory syndrome.

4. True   False   A collection of air in the pleural cavity is known as **hemothorax**.

5. True   False   The abbreviation **PND** stands for pulmonary neoplastic disease.

6. True   False   A collection of pus in the pleural cavity is known as **empyema**.

7. True   False   The abbreviation **ARDS** stands for adult research drug study.

8. True   False   A nosebleed is known as **epistaxis.**

9. True   False   The abbreviation **ABG** stands for arterial blood gases.

10. True   False   Another name for the common cold is **croup.**

11. True   False   The abbreviation **VC** stands for very critical.

12. True   False   A collection of fluid in the pleural cavity is known as **pleural effusion.**

13. True   False   The abbreviation for oxygen is **O_2.**

14. True　False　An abnormal "rice krispies" sound heard in the lungs with a stethoscope is known as **crackles**.

15. True　False　The abbreviation for carbon monoxide is CO_2.

16. True　False　**Cystic fibrosis** is a fatal genetic airway disease that causes respiratory infections and COPD in children.

17. True　False　The abbreviation **SOB** stands for short of breath.

18. True　False　**Rhonchi** is a high-pitched upper airway sound usually heard without a stethoscope, which indicates an airway obstruction.

19. True　False　The abbreviation **CPR** stands for chronic pulmonary restriction.

20. True　False　A **stat** order is to be carried out immediately.

Fill in the Blank

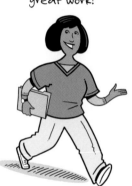

"You're over halfway there. Keep up the great work!"

Fill in the blanks below.

1. A group of diseases in which the alveolae are destroyed, resulting in chronic SOB, is ____ ____ ____ ____.

2. The disease in the question above is abbreviated

   _____.

3. Julio has _____, which causes him to become SOB and wheezy in response to various triggers.

4. A medical term for the common cold is

   _____.

5. A collection of air in the pleural cavity is known as

   _____.

6. Edelia is allergic to bees. If she gets stung, she has a severe reaction known as anaphylaxis and has great difficulty breathing. In addition to sounding wheezy, she develops a high-pitched upper airway sound caused by obstruction of her airways. This is known as

   _____.

7. When a physician gives a(n) _____ order, the expectation is that the order will be carried out immediately.

8. Sophie has a head cold. This might also be call coryza or a(n) _____ _____

   _____.

9. A skill often taught in first aid courses, which helps restore a victim's breathing and circulation, is known as

   _____ _____

   and is abbreviated _____.

10. Miguel was treated in the urgent care clinic for epistaxis. This is more commonly known as a(n) _____

    _____.

Common Diagnostic Tests

Write the definition of the following diagnostic tests.

1. **Vital capacity (VC):**

2. **Pulmonary angiography:**

3. **Arterial blood gases (ABGs):**

4. **Pulse oximetry:**

5. **Sputum analysis:**

Multiple Choice Questions

1. A coarse, gurgly sound heard with a stethoscope in the lungs, caused by secretions in the air passages, is known as:

   a. Crackles

   b. Stridor

   c. Rhonchi

   d. Wheezes

2. Which of the following tests provides an indirect measure of arterial blood oxygen saturation level?

   a. Pulse oximetry

   b. Arterial blood gases

   c. Vital capacity

   d. Sputum analysis

3. Which of the following terms indicates a condition of low oxygen?

   a. Apnea

   b. Hypoxia

   c. Dyspnea

   d. Eupnea

4. Which of the following terms means mouthlike opening in the trachea?

   a. Tracheotomy

   b. Tracheotome

   c. Tracheostomy

   d. Tracheoscopy

5. Mrs. Yachinich sleeps propped up on three pillows so she can breathe better. Which of the following terms best describes this condition?

   a. Orthopnea

   b. Aerophagia

   c. Pneumonplegia

   d. Aerophobia

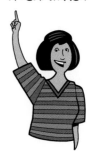

"You've completed the whole chapter. You're a real winner!"

6

DIGESTIVE SYSTEM

STRUCTURE AND FUNCTION

The digestive system is also known as the *gastrointestinal (GI) system.* It includes all structures from the mouth to the anus, including *accessory organs*. These include the pancreas, the liver, and the gallbladder, which contribute enzymes, bile, hormones, and other substances to the digestive process.

The digestive system has two key functions, *digestion* and *excretion*. We will discuss the parts of the GI system in the same order in which food passes through it. As we do this, please refer to Figure 6-1 to see the various parts of the GI system.

The first or more proximal parts of the digestive system are involved in the process of digestion. As you know, this begins in the mouth, also known as the *oral* or *buccal cavity,* when a person takes a bite of food *(ingestion)* and begins chewing it. *Mechanical digestion* occurs as food is broken down into smaller and smaller parts, mixed with *saliva,* which is secreted from three different *salivary glands* and then swallowed. As food is swallowed, it moves down a muscular tube known as the *esophagus.* It is propelled along by *peristalsis,* which is the rhythmic contraction and relaxation of the muscular wall of the esophagus. The food then enters the stomach. Mechanical digestion continues here along with the beginning of chemical digestion as the food is churned and mixed with stomach acids and enzymes.

The stomach acts as a holding tank and releases the thoroughly mixed, liquefied food, or *chyme* as it is now called, bit by bit into the *duodenum,* which is the first or most proximal portion of the small intestine.

"Peristalsis is the rhythmic muscular contractions that propel food along ... and makes your tummy growl."

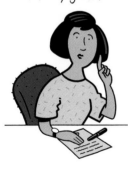

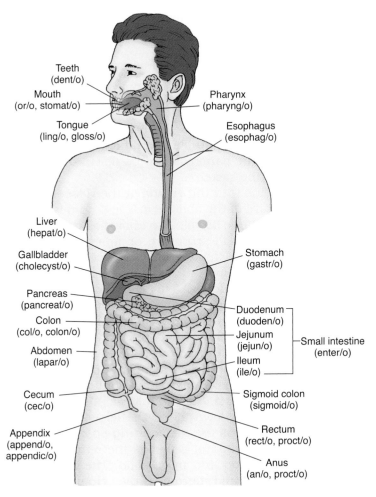

Figure 6-1 The gastrointestinal system.

It is here in the small intestine that the real action takes place. The small intestine is *small* only in the sense that it is relatively narrow; it is really quite long, around 20 feet in the average adult. Peristalsis continues to move the contents through the three parts

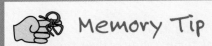

Memory Tip

It's easy to remember the correct order of the three parts of the small intestine. Just think of the phrase, "Don't juggle ice."

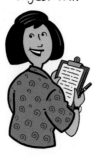

"The gallbladder stores bile, which helps digest fat."

of the small intestine: the duodenum, the **jejunum,** and the **ileum.** Here the majority of digestion is completed, and most nutrients are absorbed.

There are several accessory organs that contribute to the process of digestion. The **liver** produces **bile,** which is stored in the **gallbladder** and is secreted into the duodenum, where it **emulsifies,** or breaks down, fats. The **pancreas** secretes enzymes, which aid in digestion; the hormone **insulin,** which plays a vital role in the metabolism of proteins and fats; and **glucose,** a simple sugar. The role of the pancreas will be discussed again when we look at the endocrine system.

The jejunum joins with the **cecum** at the **ileocecal valve** in the right lower quadrant of the abdomen. The cecum is the most proximal portion of the large bowel, also known as the **colon.** Attached to the cecum is a small structure or appendage known as the **appendix.** It serves no known purpose. Occasionally, it becomes clogged with intestinal matter. As a result of the blockage, it may become inflamed and infected. This condition is known as **appendicitis.** When this occurs, the appendix must be removed by a procedure known as an **appendectomy.**

The portion of the colon that progresses upward from the cecum is known as the **ascending colon.** It takes a 90-degree turn as it nears the top of the abdomen beneath the liver and becomes the **transverse colon** as it passes horizontally across the uppermost part of the abdomen. It again takes a 90-degree turn beneath the spleen and heads down along the left side of the abdomen. This portion is known as the **descending colon.** The key function of the colon is absorption of water as the remaining waste products become less liquid and more solid. The colon then takes a gentle turn inward and becomes the **sigmoid colon,** which descends into the **rectum** and, finally, the **anus.** It is here that the intestinal contents, now a waste product known as feces, are excreted.

COMBINING FORMS

Table 6-1 contains combining forms that pertain to the digestive system, examples of medical terms that utilize the combining form, and a pronunciation guide. Read out loud to yourself as you move from left to right across the table. Be sure to use the pronunciation guide so you can learn to say the terms correctly.

TABLE 6-1

COMBINING FORMS FOR THE DIGESTIVE SYSTEM

Combining Form	Meaning	Example	Meaning of New Term
an/o	anus	anal (Ā-năl)	pertaining to the anus
append/o	appendix	appendectomy (ăp-ĕn-DĔK-tŏ-mē)	excision of the appendix
appendic/o		appendicitis (ă-pĕn-dĭ-SĪ-tĭs)	inflammation of the appendix
cholecyst/o	gallbladder	cholecystectomy (kō-lē-sĭs-TĔK-tŏ-mē)	excision of the gallbladder
col/o	colon	colectomy (kō-LĔK-tŏ-mē)	excision of the colon
colon/o		colonoscopy (kō-lŏn-ŎS-kŏ-pē)	visual examination of the colon
dent/o	teeth	dental (DĔN-tăl)	pertaining to the teeth
duoden/o	duodenum	duodenoscopy (dū-ŏd-ĕ-NŎS-kō-pē)	visual examination of the duodenum
enter/o	small intestines	enteritis (ĕn-tĕr-Ī-tĭs)	inflammation of the small intestines
esophag/o	esophagus	esophagostenosis (ē-sŏf-ă-gō-stĕn-Ō-sĭs)	narrowing of the esophagus
gastr/o	stomach	gastralgia (găs-TRĂL-jē-ă)	stomach pain
hepat/o	liver	hepatitis (hĕp-ă-TĪ-tĭs)	inflammation of the liver
ile/o	ileum	ileotomy (ĭl-ē-ŎT-ō-mē)	incision into the ileum
jenjun/o	jejunum	jejunostomy (jē-jū-NŎS-tō-mē)	mouthlike opening into the jejunum
lingu/o	tongue	sublingual (sŭb-LĬNG-gwăl)	pertaining to, beneath the tongue
gloss/o		glossospasm (GLŎS-ō-spăzm)	spasm of the tongue
lapar/o	abdomen, abdominal wall	laparoscope (LĂP-ă-rō-skōp)	an endoscope designed for visual examination of the abdominal cavity

(text continues on page 124)

COMBINING FORMS FOR THE DIGESTIVE SYSTEM (Continued)

Combining Form	Meaning	Example	Meaning of New Term
or/o	mouth	oral (ŌR-ăl)	pertaining to the mouth
stomat/o	mouth, mouthlike opening	stomatitis (stō-mă-TĪ-tĭs)	inflammation of the mouth
pancreat/o	pancreas	pancreatitis (păn-krē-ă-TĪ-tĭs)	inflammation of the pancreas
pharyng/o	pharynx	pharyngeal (făr-ĬN-jē-ăl)	pertaining to the pharynx
proct/o	rectum anus	proctoscopy (prŏk-TŎS-kŏ-pē)	visual examination of the rectum and anus
rect/o	rectum	rectal (RĔK-tăl)	pertaining to the rectum
sigmoid/o	sigmoid colon	sigmoidoscope (sĭg-MOY-dō-skōp)	instrument used to examine the sigmoid colon

STOP HERE.

Select the Combining Form Flash Cards for Chapter 6, and run through them at least 3 times before you continue.

PRACTICE EXERCISE

Use Table 6-1 to fill in the answers below.

1. _____ pertaining to the rectum

2. _____ an endoscope designed for visual examination of the abdominal cavity

3. _____ pertaining to the mouth

4. _____ pertaining to the pharynx

5. _____ pertaining to the anus

6. _____ narrowing of the esophagus

7. _____ excision of the gallbladder

8. _____ inflammation of the small
intestines

9. _____ mouthlike opening into the
jejunum

10. _____ visual examination of the colon

11. _____ pertaining to, beneath the tongue

12. _____ visual examination of the
duodenum

13. _____ incision into the ileum

14. _____ inflammation of the mouth

15. _____ stomach pain

16. _____ inflammation of the liver

17. _____ excision of the appendix

18. _____ inflammation of the appendix

19. _____ visual examination of the rectum
and anus

20. _____ excision of the colon

21. _____ pertaining to the teeth

22. _____ spasm of the tongue

23. _____ inflammation of the pancreas

24. _____ instrument used to examine the
sigmoid colon

25. Fill in the blanks with the appropriate anatomical term and/or combining form.

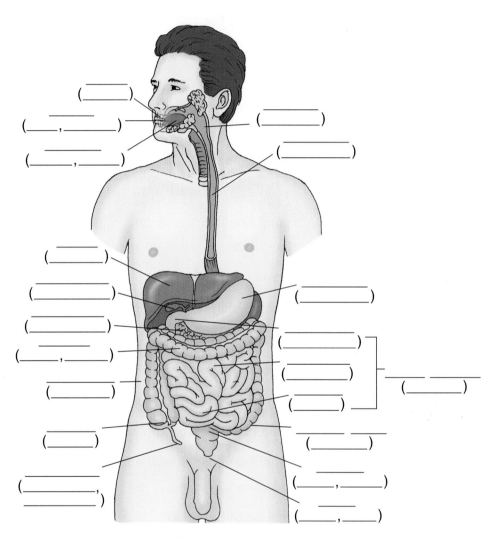

Figure 6-2

ABBREVIATIONS

Table 6-2 lists some of the most common abbreviations related to the GI system as well as others often used in medical documentation.

TABLE 6-2
ABBREVIATIONS

Abd	abdomen
BRP	bathroom privileges
BM	bowel movement
c̄	with
c/o	complain(s,t) of,
CA	cancer
Dx	diagnosis
EGD	esophagogastroduodenoscopy
ERCP	endoscopic retrograde cholangiopancreatography
GERD	gastroesophageal reflux disease
GI	gastrointestinal
hr, h	hour
IBD	inflammatory bowel disease
IBS	irritable bowel syndrome
LFT	liver function test
NG	nasogastric
N&V	nausea and vomiting
NPO	nothing by mouth
PO	by mouth
PR	per rectum
PUD	peptic ulcer disease
q	every
SBO	small bowel obstruction
s̄	without
UGI	upper gastrointestinal
VS	vital signs

STOP HERE.
Select the Abbreviation Flash Cards for Chapter 6, and run through them at least 3 times before you continue.

PATHOLOGY TERMS

Table 6-3 includes terms that relate to diseases or abnormalities of the digestive system. Use the pronunciation guide, and say the terms out loud as you read them. This will help you get in the habit of saying them properly.

TABLE 6-3
PATHOLOGY TERMS

ascites (ă-SĪ-tēz)	accumulation of serous fluid in the peritoneal (abdominal) cavity
bowel obstruction (BOW-ĕl)	a partial or complete blockage of the small or large intestine; common causes include volvulus, intussusception, tumors, and adhesions (scar tissue)
cirrhosis (sĭ-RŌ-sĭs)	a chronic liver disease characterized by scarring and loss of normal structure
diverticulosis (dī-vĕr-tĭk-ū-LŌ-sĭs)	a condition in which small pouches (diverticula) form in the intestinal wall, due to increased pressure (Fig. 6-3)
diverticulitis (dī-vĕr-tĭk-ū-LĪ-tĭs)	when one or more diverticula become inflamed (see Fig. 6-3)
emesis (ĔM-ĕ-sĭs)	vomiting
hernia (HĔR-nē-ă)	the protrusion of a structure through the wall that normally contains it
intussusception (ĭn-tŭ-sŭ-SĔP-shŭn)	the slipping or telescoping of a portion of the bowel into itself (Fig. 6-4)
irritable bowel syndrome	chronic condition characterized by alternating episodes of constipation and diarrhea
jaundice (JAWN-dĭs)	a condition marked by yellow staining of body tissues and fluids as a result of excessive levels of bilirubin in the blood
peptic ulcer (PĔP-tĭk ŬL-sĕr)	an inflamed lesion in the gastric or duodenal lining
volvulus (VŎL-vū-lŭs)	a twisting of the bowel upon itself, causing obstruction (Fig. 6-5)
ulcerative colitis (ŬL-sĕr-ā-tĭv kō-LĪ-tĭs)	chronic inflammatory disease of the lining of the colon marked by up to 20 liquid bloody stools per day
Crohn's disease (krōnz dĭ-ZĒZ)	an inflammatory bowel disease marked by patches of full-thickness inflammation anywhere in the GI tract

"When it comes to pronunciations, there is only one word for you: practice."

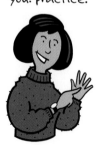

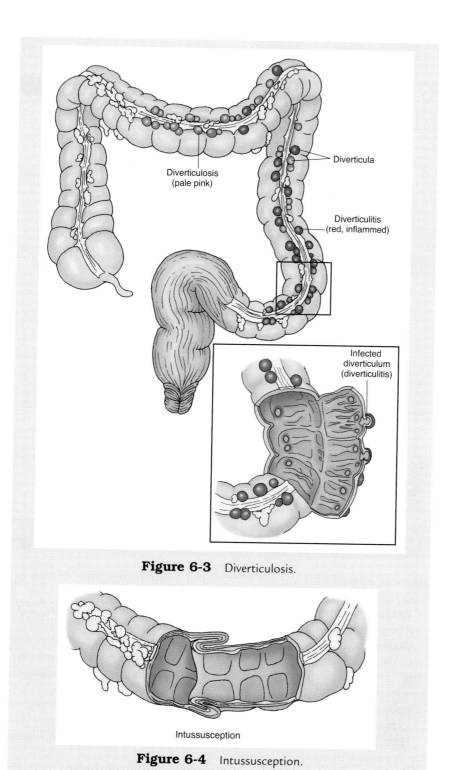

Figure 6-3 Diverticulosis.

Diverticulosis
(pale pink)

Diverticula

Diverticulitis
(red, inflammed)

Infected
diverticulum
(diverticulitis)

Intussusception

Figure 6-4 Intussusception.

(text continues on page 130)

129

PATHOLOGY TERMS *(Continued)*

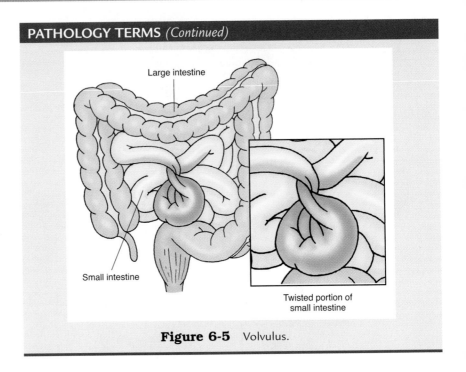

Large intestine

Small intestine

Twisted portion of
small intestine

Figure 6-5   Volvulus.

STOP HERE.
Select the Pathology Terms Flash Cards for Chapter 6, and
run through them at least 3 times before you continue.

COMMON DIAGNOSTIC TESTS

Barium enema: An enema containing a substance that shows up
well under x-ray and fluoroscopic examination.

Barium swallow: An x-ray examination of the esophagus after
the patient swallows a liquid that contains barium.

Computed tomography (CT) scan: Computerized collection
and translation of multiple x-rays into a three-dimensional picture; creates a more detailed and accurate image than traditional
x-rays (Fig. 6-6)

Gastroccult: gastric contents are tested for the presence of
blood and pH level

Hemoccult (stool guaiac test): small sample of feces is tested
for presence of blood

Endoscopic retrograde cholangiopancreatography (ERCP):
radiographic examination of vessels that connect the liver, gallbladder, and pancreas to the duodenum after a radiopaque material is injected though a fiberoptic endoscope

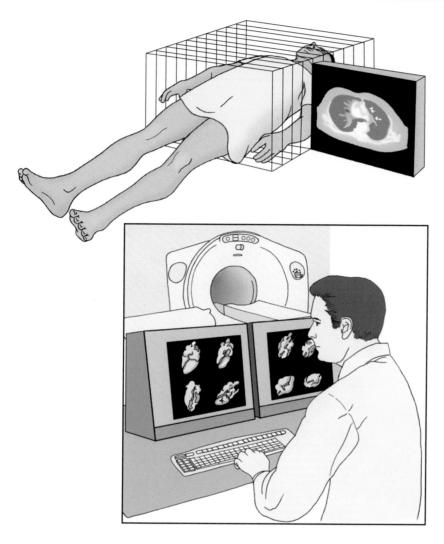

Figure 6-6 Computed tomography scan.

Laparoscopy: exploration of the contents of the abdomen using a laparoscope

Lower endoscopy: visual examination of the GI tract, from rectum to cecum (Fig. 6-7)

Stool culture: sample of feces is examined for presence of bacteria and other microorganisms

Ultrasound: ultra-high frequency sound waves are used to outline the shape of various structures in the body

Upper endoscopy: visual examination of the GI tract, from esophagus to duodenum (Fig. 6-8)

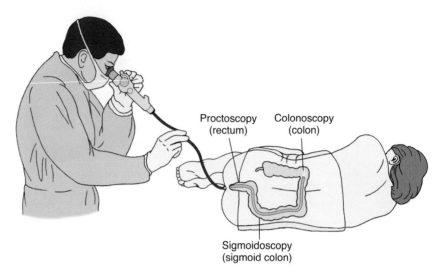

Figure 6-7 Lower endoscopy (proctoscopy, sigmoidoscopy, colonoscopy).

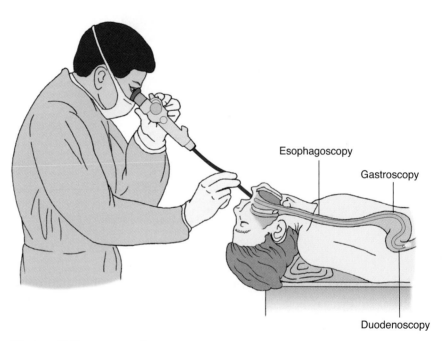

Figure 6-8 Upper endoscopy (esophagoscopy, gastroscopy, duodenoscopy).

CASE STUDY

"You may very well see
patients like Cynthia
when you enter
practice."

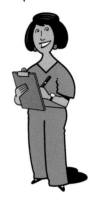

Read the following case study, and answer the questions that follow. Most of the terms are included in this chapter. Refer to the Glossary or to your medical dictionary for the other terms.

Ulcerative Colitis

Cynthia Summers is a 34-year-old married woman with two small children. She was seen by a physician at Valley Clinic this morning for an exacerbation of her ulcerative colitis. Her chief complaints were of three to five episodes of bloody diarrhea per day, cramping abdominal pain, and fatigue. Cynthia was thin and pale. She appeared anxious and was reluctant to go to the hospital, stating that she needed to go home to take care of her family.

The physician prescribed prednisone and gave her the following dietary recommendations: eat high-calorie foods, avoid strong spices or caffeine, and drink plenty of fluids. She is to return in 3 days for a follow-up visit or sooner if her condition worsens. If her condition cannot be controlled with medications and dietary changes, hospitalization and possible surgery will be considered.

Ulcerative colitis is characterized by chronic inflammation of the large intestine, primarily the rectum and sigmoid colon. Onset is usually in a patient's early 20s. Lesions form in the mucosal layer, causing very tiny hemorrhages that may, in time, develop abscesses. The lesions may become necrotic and ulcerate. The primary symptom of ulcerative colitis is bloody diarrhea accompanied by cramping abdominal pain. Episodes of diarrhea may vary from once or twice a day to as many as 30 to 40 times a day in very severe cases. As a result, anorexia, anemia, and fatigue are common. The disease usually has periods of exacerbation and remissions. Treatment includes steroid medication such as prednisone, which has a powerful anti-inflammatory effect, and dietary modifications. Severe cases may require surgical intervention in which part or all of the colon is removed (partial or complete colectomy). People with ulcerative colitis have an increased risk for developing colon cancer.

Case Study Questions

1. Ulcerative colitis usually affects which part of the intestine?
   a. Ileum
   b. Jejunum
   c. Proximal colon
   d. Distal colon

(continues on page 134)

2. The medication the physician prescribed should help Cynthia because:
   a. It is an analgesic, which reduces pain
   b. It is an antibiotic, which will promote healing
   c. It will reduce inflammation in her colon
   d. It reduces pain by reducing acids in the intestine

3. The age of onset of ulcerative colitis is usually:
   a. In childhood
   b. In the early 20s
   c. In the 40s
   d. After age 60

4. Lesions may become abscessed, which means that they:
   a. Become infected
   b. Bleed
   c. Swell
   d. Contain dead tissue

5. The lesions may eventually become necrotic, which means that they:
   a. Heal
   b. Contain dead tissue
   c. Swell
   d. Bleed

6. In severe cases of ulcerative colitis, the patient experiences:
   a. Weight gain
   b. Constipation
   c. Frequent nausea
   d. Loss of appetite

7. Ulcerative colitis is characterized by:
   a. Periods of improvement alternating with periods of worsening
   b. Sudden, acute onset; short duration; and total healing
   c. Gradual onset, lengthy illness, and eventual complete healing
   d. Gradual onset, chronic disability. and eventual death

WEB SITES

American Liver Foundation: www.liverfoundation.org
American Dental Association: www.ADA.org

PREFIX AND SUFFIX REVIEW

Tables 6-4 and 6-5 contain a review of selected prefixes and suffixes. Refer to these tables if necessary when you complete the exercises at the end of the chapter.

TABLE 6-4
PREFIX PRONUNCIATIONS AND MEANINGS

Prefix	Pronunciation Guide	Meaning
a-	ā	without, absence of
circum-	sĕr-kŭm	around
dys-	dĭs	painful, difficult
hyper-	hī-pĕr	excessive, above normal
hypo- sub-	hī-pō, sŭb	below normal, beneath
micro-	mī-krō	small
peri-	pĕr-ĭ	near, surrounding

TABLE 6-5
SUFFIX PRONUNCIATIONS AND MEANINGS

Suffix	Pronunciation Guide	Meaning
-al, -ic	ăl,	pertaining to
-algia -dynia	ăl-jē-ă dĭn-ē-ă	pain
-ectomy	ĕk-tō-mē	excision, surgical removal
-emesis	ĕm-ĕ-sĭs	vomiting
-itis	ī-tĭs	inflammation
-kinesia	kĭ-nē-sĭs	movement

(continues on page 136)

SUFFIX PRONUNCIATIONS AND MEANINGS *(Continued)*

Suffix	Pronunciation Guide	Meaning
-lith	lĭth	stone
-logist	lō-jĭst	specialist in the study of
-logy	lō-jē	study of
-malacia	mă-lā-sē-ă	softening
-megaly	mĕg-ă-lē	enlargement
-oma	ō-mă	tumor
-osis	ō-sĭs	abnormal condition
-paresis	păr-ē-sĭs	slight or partial paralysis
-pathy	pă-thē	disease
-pepsia	pĕp-sē-ă	digestion
-phagia	fā-jē-ă	eating, swallowing
-phasia	fā-zē-ă	speech
-phoria	fō-rē-ă	feeling
-plasty	plăs-tē	surgical repair
-plegia	plē-jē-ă	paralysis
-rrhea	rē-ă	flow, discharge
-scope	skōp	instrument to view
-scopy	skō-pē	visual examination
-stenosis	stĕ-nō-sĭs	narrowing, stricture
-stomy	stō-mē	mouthlike opening
-tomy	tō-mē	cutting into, incision
-tripsy	trĭp-sē	crushing
-trophy	trō-fē	nourishment or growth

PRACTICE EXERCISES

Complete the following practice exercises. The answers can be found in Appendix G.

"Checking your answers AFTER you've completed these exercises provides immediate feedback that will reinforce your learning."

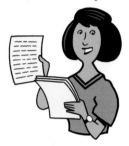

Matching

Match the following prefixes with the correct meanings. Some answers may be used more than once or not at all.

Exercise A

1. _____ or/o

2. _____ proct/o

3. _____ jejun/o

4. _____ enter/o

5. _____ appendic/o

6. _____ hepat/o

7. _____ stomat/o

8. _____ dent/o

9. _____ append/o

10. _____ lingu/o

a. appendix

b. small intestine

c. stomach

d. tongue

e. teeth

f. mouth or mouthlike structure

g. ileum

h. jejunum

i. rectum or anus

j. liver

Exercise B

1. _____ col/o

2. _____ cholecyst/o

3. _____ an/o

4. _____ ile/o

a. rectum

b. pharynx

c. liver

d. colon

5. _____ rect/o   e. sigmoid colon

6. _____ sigmoid/o   f. gallbladder

7. _____ pharyng/o   g. duodenum

8. _____ pancreat/o   h. anus

9. _____ duoden/o   i. pancreas

10. _____ colon/o   j. ileum

Word Building

*Using **only** the word parts in the lists provided, create medical terms with the indicated meanings.*

Prefixes	Combining Forms	Suffixes
circum-	an/o	-al
hyper-	append/o	-ectomy
hypo-	chol/e	-emesis
peri-	cholecyst/o	-ic
	colon/o	-itis
	dent/o	-lith
	esophag/o	-megaly
	gastr/o	-oma
	hepat/o	-scopy
	ile/o	-stomy
	or/o	-tomy
	jejun/o	-pathy

1. Disease of the liver _____

2. Inflammation of the esophagus _____

3. Visual examination of the esophagus and
   stomach _____

4. Pertaining to around the mouth _____

5. Excision and removal of the
   gallbladder _____

6. Enlarged stomach _____

7. Pertaining to above the large intestine _____

8. Pertaining to the area near the anus _____

9. Mouthlike opening into the jejunum. _____

10. A tumor of the liver _____

11. Inflammation of the appendix _____

12. Excision or removal of the appendix _____

13. Incision into the ileum _____

14. Excessive vomiting _____

15. Pertaining to the teeth _____

16. Inflammation of the gallbladder _____

17. Pertaining to below or beneath the
    stomach _____

18. Visual examination of the large
    intestine _____

19. A bile stone _____

20. Disease of the large intestine _____

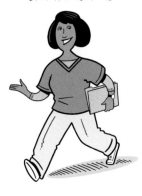

"You're off to a great start. Fabulous!"

Deciphering Terms

Write the correct translation of the following medical terms.

1. cholecystectomy _____

2. enteritis _____

3. proctoscopy _____

4. gastroscope _____

5. laparoscopy _____

6. jejunoplasty _____

7. pancreatolith _____

8. sublingual _____

9. pharyngitis _____

10. gastroenterologist _____

11. microgastric _____

12. dyskinesia _____

13. diarrhea _____

14. gastroparesis _____

15. dysphoria _____

16. atrophy _____

17. proctology _____

18. lithotripsy _____

19. dyspepsia _____

20. oralgia _____

True or False

Decide whether the following statements are true or false.

1. True   False   The abbreviation **s̄** means "with."

2. True   False   The abbreviation **q** stands for every.

3. True   False   **Crohn's disease** is a chronic inflammatory disease of the lining of the colon, marked by up to 20 liquid bloody stools per day.

4. True   False   The abbreviation **LFT** stands for liver function test.

5. True   False   **Irritable bowel syndrome** is a chronic condition characterized by alternating episodes of constipation and diarrhea.

6. True   False   The abbreviation **PUD** stands for peptic ulcer disease.

7. True   False   An **EGD** is a procedure that involves examination of the liver.

8. True   False   The abbreviation **BM** stands for basal metabolic rate.

9. True   False   An accumulation of fluid in the peritoneal cavity is known as **cirrhosis.**

10. True   False   The abbreviation **GI** stands for gastrointestinal.

11. True   False   The abbreviation **GERD** stands for gastroesophageal reflux disease.

12. True   False   The abbreviation **IBS** stands for intestinal blockage syndrome.

13. True   False   A **volvulus** occurs when the bowel twists on itself, causing obstruction.

14. True   False   If the physician has ordered a medication to be administered **NG,** it means it will be given through a nasogastic tube.

15. True   False   The abbreviation **VS** stands for very serious.

16. True   False   The protrusion of a structure through the wall that normally contains it is known as a **hernia.**

17. True   False   The abbreviation **h** stands for help.

18. True   False   An inflamed lesion in the stomach or duodenal lining is known as a **peptic ulcer.**

19. True   False   The abbreviation **d** stands for day.

Fill in the Blank

Fill in the blanks below.

1. _____ is the *accumulation of serous fluid in the peritoneal cavity.*

2. A condition in which *small pouches form in the intestinal wall* is _____.

3. When the condition in the question above becomes inflamed, it is known as _____.

4. The abbreviation *ERCP* stands for _____ _____ _____ _____.

5. Another term for *vomiting* is _____.

6. The abbreviation _____ means *with.*

7. A *chronic disease of the colon marked by inflammation and frequent bloody diarrhea* is _____.

8. The *abdomen* may be abbreviated as _____.

9. The abbreviation *UGI* stands for _____ _____ _____.

10. The abbreviation *SBO* stands for _____ _____ _____.

11. If a patient is *not to eat or drink anything,* the physician may write this order: _____.

12. If a medication is to be taken *orally,* the order will be _____.

13. A suppository medication that is given *rectally* may be ordered _____.

"You're doing great! keep going!"

14. If *vital signs are to be taken once every hour*, the physician may write the following order: "_____ _____ _____."

15. If a patient is to be weighed *every day*, the physician may write the following order: "weigh _____ _____".

16. When *a portion of the bowel slips inside of itself*, it is called

    _____.

17. *Excessive levels of bilirubin in the blood may result in yellow staining of body tissues.* This is known as

    _____.

18. _____ is the abbreviation for cancer.

19. A physician writes the following order: "*Bedrest with bathroom privileges.*" How might this order be abbreviated?

    _____.

20. The physician dictates that the patient "*c/o N&V*". This means that the patient _____.

Common Diagnostic Tests

Write the definition of the following diagnostic tests.

1. **Barium enema:**

2. **Barium swallow:**

3. **Computed tomography (CT) scan:**

4. **Endoscopic retrograde cholangiopancreatography (ERCP):**

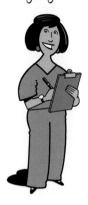

"You learn by repetition, so keep going!"

5. **Gastroccult:**

6. **Hemoccult (stool guaiac test):**

7. **Laparoscopy:**

8. **Lower endoscopy:**

9. **Stool culture:**

10. **Ultrasound:**

11. **Upper endoscopy:**

Multiple Choice Questions

Select the one best answer to the following multiple choice questions.

1. Mr. Green is a 63-year-old man with heartburn (GERD). When it flares up, he experiences:

   a. Gastromegaly

   b. Esophagoplegia

   c. Esophagodynia

   d. Gastromalacia

2. Mr. Smith, a 36-year-old man, has come to the clinic complaining of symptoms that are consistent with heartburn (GERD). Which of the following procedures will accurately diagnose this condition?

   a. Laparoscopy

   b. Upper endoscopy

   c. Esophogectomy

   d. Enteropathy

3. Ms. Diaz is a 47-year-old woman with a bowel obstruction. It is caused by a portion of her bowel twisting upon itself. This condition is known as:

   a. Intussusception

   b. Ulcerative colitis

   c. Volvulus

   d. Cirrhosis

4. Mr. Washington, a 27-year-old man, has a sore throat due to inflammation. Which of the following is the correct medical term for this condition?

   a. Pharyngitis

   b. Pharyngostenosis

   c. Colitis

   d. Stomatitis

5. Which of the following terms is NOT related to a part of the small intestine?

   a. Duoden/o

   b. Jujen/o

   c. Colon/o

   d. Ile/o

6. Which of the following terms means "difficult or painful swallowing"?

   a. Dyspepsia

   b. Dysphagia

   c. Dysphasia

   d. Dysphoria

"You've completed the entire chapter. What a great accomplishment!"

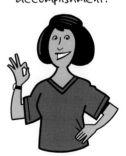

7 URINARY SYSTEM

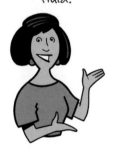

STRUCTURE AND FUNCTION

The key organs of the urinary system are the **kidneys,** which are located in the back of the abdominal cavity in the **retroperitoneal space** (Fig. 7-1). The kidneys are responsible for several important functions in the body but are most commonly known for their role in filtering blood.

The functional unit of the kidneys where most of the action takes place is a microscopic structure known as the **nephron** (Fig. 7-2). There are approximately one million nephrons in each kidney. The nephron contains a filtration unit called the glomerulus, which encloses a tiny round cluster of capillaries. This is where the process of filtration begins as fluid and wastes are removed from the blood.

Once the filtered fluid leaves the glomerulus, it passes through the tubules of the nephron, where adjustments are made in the final amount of water and *electrolytes* (such as sodium and potassium) that will be excreted. The end product, known as *urine*, then drains from each kidney down a long, narrow tube called a *ureter* and collects in the *urinary bladder.*

When the volume of urine in the bladder reaches a certain level, stretch receptors in the bladder wall are stimulated, which results in the **micturition reflex.** This is the familiar urge we get to empty our bladder. This urge can be ignored temporarily, but eventually the stretch receptors will be stimulated again, and the urge to **urinate,** or **void,** will be even stronger. A classic example of this is the small child who is too busy playing to heed this urge until it becomes too strong too deny. Then there is a mad dash for the nearest bathroom. As the bladder empties, the urine passes out through another narrow tubelike structure known as the **urethra.**

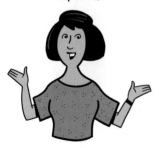

"But the real action happens in the nephrons."

146

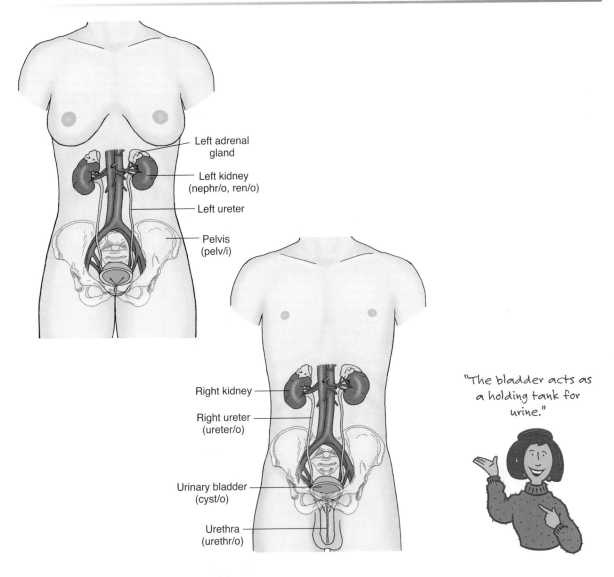

Left adrenal gland

Left kidney (nephr/o, ren/o)

Left ureter

Pelvis (pelv/i)

Right kidney

Right ureter (ureter/o)

Urinary bladder (cyst/o)

Urethra (urethr/o)

"The bladder acts as a holding tank for urine."

Figure 7-1 The urinary system.

The urethra is less than an inch long in women and several inches long in men.

In addition to filtering fluid and wastes from the body, the kidneys play an active role in maintaining blood pressure. They do this by regulating fluid volume as well as electrolyte levels.

Another important function of the kidneys is maintenance of blood **pH.** This reflects how acidic or alkaline the blood is on the pH scale. Even though the entire acid-base scale ranges from

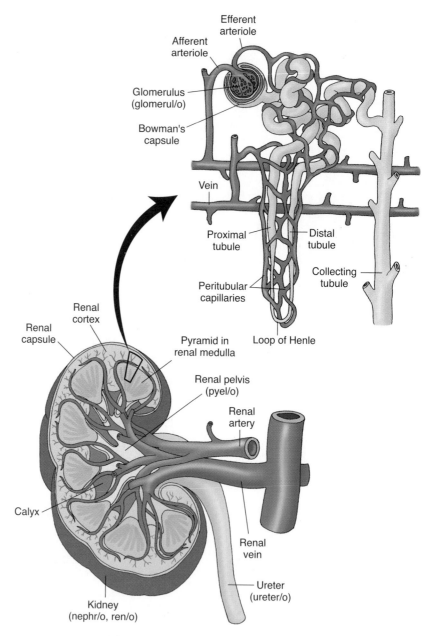

Figure 7-2   The kidney and the nephron.

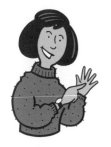

"The pH scale goes from 0 to 14 ..."

0 to 14, the pH of blood in the human body must remain slightly alkaline within the very narrow range of 7.35 to 7.45. Even minor fluctuations in this balance will result in illness or even death. So as you can see, the kidneys are extremely important to the maintenance of homeostasis.

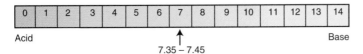

0	1	2	3	4	5	6	7	8	9	10	11	12	13	14

Acid   Base

↑
7.35 – 7.45

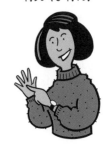

" ... but our blood must stay in the very narrow range of 7.35 to 7.45."

Occasionally, a person may have kidney failure, also known as **renal failure.** A common cause is the destructive effects of poorly controlled **diabetes.** This is a disorder of the pancreas in which insulin is not properly excreted or utilized, resulting in abnormal **glucose** (sugar) and fat metabolism. This disorder is discussed more thoroughly in Chapter 9, The Endocrine System.

In some cases when a person has renal failure, he or she is able to receive a kidney **transplant.** You may have heard of situations in which one person donates a kidney to another person. This illustrates two important points: one is that most people can live a long and normal life with only one healthy kidney; the other is that it is very difficult to lead a long and normal life without any kidneys at all.

If the person is not able to receive a transplant, he or she may live for months or even years by having regular **hemodialysis.** This is a process in which the blood is filtered through a special membrane in a dialysis machine to remove excess fluid and wastes (Fig. 7-3).

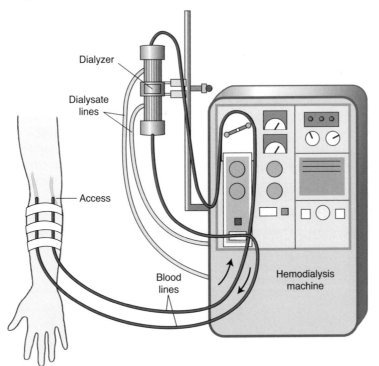

"In hemodialysis, the patient is hooked up to a machine that filters wastes and excess fluid from the blood."

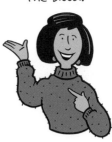

Figure 7-3 Hemodialysis.

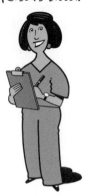

"With peritoneal dialysis, a fluid, called dialysate, is instilled into the person's abdomen. It is later drained out along with the wastes that were removed from that person's blood."

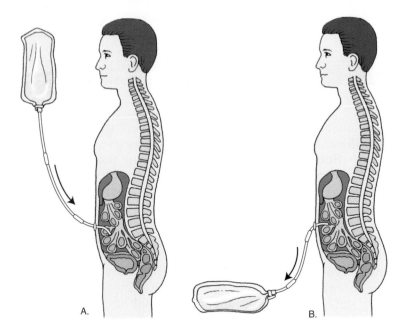

A.

B.

Figure 7-4   Peritoneal dialysis.

Another type of dialysis, in which the patient is not hooked up to a machine, is known as **peritoneal** dialysis. In this case, the patient's own peritoneal membrane in his or her abdominal cavity is used as a filter (Fig. 7-4).

COMBINING FORMS

Tables 7-1 and 7-2 contain combining forms that pertain to the urinary system, examples of terms that utilize the combining form, and a pronunciation guide. Read out loud to yourself as you move from left to right across the table. Be sure to use the pronunciation guide so that you can learn to say the terms correctly.

TABLE 7-1
COMBINING FORMS RELATED TO THE URINARY SYSTEM

Combining Form	Meaning	Example	Meaning of New Term
cyst/o	bladder	cystoscopy (sĭs-TŎS-kō-pē)	visual examination of the bladder
glomerul/o	glomerulus	glomerulopathy (glō-mĕr-ū-LŎP-ă-thē)	disease of the glomerulus

Combining Form	Meaning	Example	Meaning of New Term
nephr/o	kidney	nephrologist (ně-FRŎL-ō-jĭst)	specialist in the study of the kidneys
ren/o		renal (RĒ-năl)	pertaining to the kidneys
pyel/o	renal pelvis	pyelonephritis (pī-ě-lō-ně-FRĪ-tĭs)	inflammation (infection) of the renal pelvis and kidney
ureter/o	ureter	ureterostenosis (ū-rē-těr-ō-stě-NŌ-sĭs)	narrowing or stricture of the ureter
urethr/o	urethra	urethropexy (ū-RĒ-thrō-pěks-ē)	surgical fixation of the urethra
ur/o	urine	urology (ū-RŎL-ō-jē)	study of disorders of the urinary tract
urin/o		urinometer (ū-rĭ-NŎM-ě-těr)	instrument for measuring urine

TABLE 7-2
OTHER COMBINING FORMS

Combining Form	Meaning	Example	Meaning of New Term
bacteri/o	bacteria	bacteriuria (băk-tē-rē-Ū-rē-ă)	bacteria in the urine
hemat/o	blood	hematuria (hē-mă-TŪ-rē-ă)	blood in the urine
hem/o		hemolysis (hē-MŎL-ĭ-sĭs)	destruction of blood
lith/o	stone	nephrolithiasis (něf-rō-lĭth-Ī-ă-sĭs)	abnormal condition of kidney stones
noct/o	night	nocturia (nŏk-TŪ-rē-ă)	urination at night
olig/o	deficient	oliguria (ōl-ĭg-Ū-rē-ă)	deficiency of urine
peritine/o	peritoneum	peritoneal (pěr-ĭ-tō-NĒ-ăl)	pertaining to the peritoneum
py/o	pus	pyuria (pī-Ū-rē-ă)	pus in the urine

"Notice that many of the combining forms in Table 7-2 are paired with the suffix -uria to describe abnormalities of the urine."

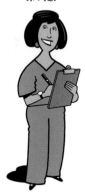

 ## STOP HERE.
Remove the Combining Forms Flash Cards for Chapter 7, and run through them at least 3 times before you continue.

PRACTICE EXERCISES

Use Tables 7-1 and 7-2 to fill in the answers below.

1. _____ pertaining to the peritoneum

2. _____ urination at night

3. _____ blood in the urine

4. _____ bacteria in the urine

5. _____ surgical fixation of the urethra

6. _____ inflammation (infection) of the renal pelvis and kidney

7. _____ disease of the glomerulus

8. _____ visual examination of the bladder

9. _____ destruction of blood

10. _____ specialist in the study of the kidneys

11. _____ narrowing or stricture of the ureter

12. _____ study of disorders of the urinary tract

13. _____ instrument for measuring urine

14. _____ abnormal condition of kidney stones

15. _____ deficiency of urine

16. _____ pus in the urine

17. _____ pertaining to the kidneys

18. Fill in the blanks with the appropriate anatomical term and/or combining form.

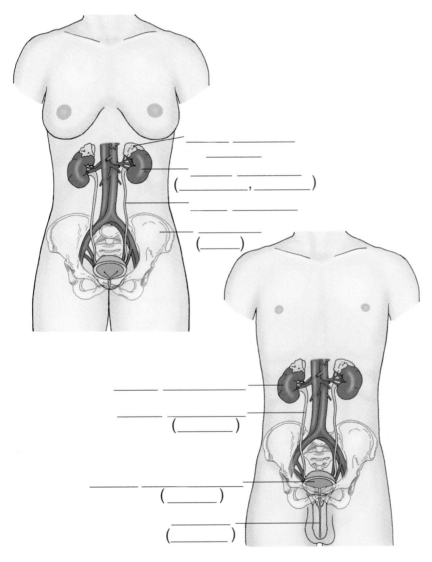

Figure 7-5

19. Fill in the blanks with the appropriate anatomical term and/or combining form.

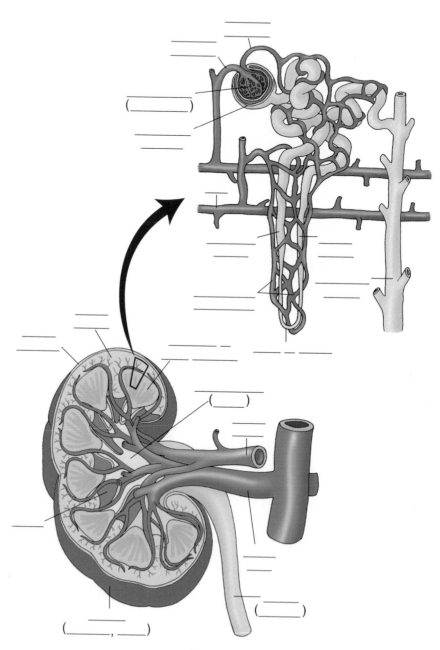

Figure 7-6

ABBREVIATIONS

Table 7-3 lists some of the most common abbreviations related to the urinary system as well as others often used in medical documentation.

TABLE 7-3	
ABBREVIATIONS	
BPH	benign prostatic hypertrophy (benign prostatic hyperplasia)
ESRD	end-stage renal disease
IVP	intravenous pyelogram
KUB	kidney, ureter, bladder
RP	retrograde pyelogram
TURP	transurethral resection of the prostate
UA	urinalysis
UTI	urinary tract infection

STOP HERE.
Remove the Abbreviations Flash Cards for Chapter 7, and run through them at least 3 times before you continue.

 Memory Tip

A TURP is a procedure done to relieve the symptoms caused by an enlarged prostate (BPH). Remember this relationship by connecting the two abbreviations in the following manner:

      B
TURP
      H

PATHOLOGY TERMS

Table 7-4 includes terms that relate to diseases or abnormalities of the urinary system. Use the pronunciation guide and say the terms out loud as you read them. This will help you get in the habit of saying them properly.

TABLE 7-4

PATHOLOGY TERMS

diuresis (dī-ū-RĒ-sĭs)	abnormal secretion of large amounts of urine
end-stage renal disease (ESRD)	final phase of kidney disease
enuresis (ĕn-ū-RĒ-sĭs)	involuntary urination during sleep; also called bed-wetting
glycosuria (glĭ-kō-SŪ-rē-ă) **glucosuria** (gloo-kō-SŪ-rē-ă)	sugar in the urine
interstitial nephritis (ĭn-tĕr-STĬSH-ăl nĕf-RĪ-tĭs)	pathological changes in renal tissue that destroy nephrons and impair kidney function
interstitial cystitis (ĭn-tĕr-STĬSH-ăl sĭs-TĪ-tĭs)	chronic condition of inflammation of the bladder lining
phimosis (fī-MŌ-sĭs)	stenosis or narrowing of the foreskin opening (Fig. 7-7)

Phimosis

Figure 7-7 Phimosis.

pyelonephritis (pī-ĕ-lō-nĕ-FRĪ-tĭs)	inflammation and infection caused by bacterial growth in the renal pelvis and kidney
renal failure	failure of the kidneys to effectively eliminate fluids and/or wastes from the body
stress incontinence	involuntary urine leakage upon physical stress, such as a cough or sneeze
urinary retention	retention of urine in the bladder due to an inability to urinate
urinary tract infection (UTI)	inflammation and infection caused by bacterial growth in the urinary tract, usually the bladder
uremia (ū-RĒ-mē-ă)	increased level of urea or other wastes in the blood

STOP HERE.
Remove the Pathology Term Flash Cards for Chapter 7, and run through them at least 3 times before you continue.

Memory Tip

Remember the difference in the meaning of the following terms by using the associations shown below.

diuresis happens in the **d**aytime (usually) in response to **d**rugs

enuresis happens **en** (in) bed while you sleep

nocturia wakes you up at **n**ight

"I sure wish these memory tips were around when I was in school!"

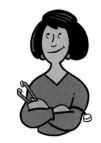

COMMON DIAGNOSTIC TESTS

Blood urea nitrogen (BUN): A lab value used to measure kidney function based on nitrogen levels in the blood

Culture and sensitivity (C&S): Growing microorganisms, then exposing them to antimicrobial drugs to determine which drugs kill them most effectively

24-hour urine specimen: total urine excreted over 24 hours is collected for analysis

Intravenous pyelogram (IVP): X-ray examination of the kidneys, ureters, and bladder after injection of a contrast medium

Serum creatinine: A lab value used to measure kidney function; more specific than BUN

Urinalysis (UA): Visual and microscopic analysis of a urine specimen (Table 7-5)

TABLE 7-5		
NORMAL VALUES OF A URINALYSIS		
Chem Stick		Microscopic
Color	Lt yellow or straw	Epithelial Cells: 3-4
Appearance	Clear	WBCs: 0-1
S.G.	1.010–1.030	RBCs: 0
pH	5-8	Bacteria: 0
Protein	neg	
Glucose	neg	
Ketones	neg	
Bilirubin	neg	
Blood:	neg	
Nitrites	neg	

CASE STUDY

Read the following case study and answer the questions that follow. Most of the terms are included in this chapter. Refer to the Glossary or to your medical dictionary for the other terms.

Interstitial Cystitis

Lisa is a 32-year-old woman who came to her nurse practitioner 2 months ago with c/o frequency, urgency, dysuria, and low back and pelvic pain. A urine specimen was collected and analyzed. The findings were normal except for a small number of RBCs. Because of her symptoms, she was treated for a possible UTI and was put on a course of antibiotics. She returned a week later with her symptoms unchanged. A second urine specimen was tested, with the same results as the first time. Then Lisa was put on a different antibiotic. When she returned a week later, with still no improvement in Sx, she was referred to a urologist for further evaluation.

After an initial consultation with the urologist, a cystoscopy was done under general anesthesia, and tissue was collected for a Bx. The cytology report revealed that the specimen was benign. However, visual inspection during the cystoscopy confirmed the presence of hemorrhagic lesions and ulcerations as well as smaller-than-normal bladder capacity. Based on these findings a Dx of interstitial cystitis was confirmed. A bladder distention was performed at that time.

Interstitial cystitis (IC) is an uncommon disorder affecting approximately 500,000 people in the United States; 90% of those affected are women. The cause has not been clearly identified, although severe stress appears to be a contributor. There is also some speculation that it may be autoimmune in nature as well. There is no known cure. Treatments are few and provide variable results.

People with IC manage their disease most effectively by noticing what seems to trigger or worsen their symptoms and what brings relief. It is essentially a process of trial and error; the results are not the same for everyone. Some dietary triggers may include caffeine, alcohol, chocolate, and acidic foods such as citrus fruits. Therefore, the usual remedy of drinking cranberry juice for a bladder infection is **not** helpful and may exacerbate Sx. Some interventions that may bring relief include taking Elmiron (the only medication approved so far for IC), taking nonsteroidal anti-inflammatory drugs (NSAIDs) such as ibuprofen or naproxen, and applying heat. People with IC generally notice wide fluctuations in Sx and will have good days and bad days. They may need to adopt lifestyle modifications and avoid activities that seem to increase their pain.

Common symptoms of IC include low back and pelvic pain, **frequency** (the need to urinate often, caused by bladder irritation), **urgency** (the need to urinate *now*), and **dysuria** (pain or burning on urination). The symptoms are extremely variable in duration and intensity and may fluctuate dramatically throughout any given day.

Definitive diagnosis is done via cystoscopy, which may be done under general anesthesia if bladder distention is planned. In this procedure, the bladder is filled with sterile saline to stretch it and increase its capacity.

Case Study Questions

1. Lisa initially presented to her nurse practitioner with which of the following symptoms?
   a. Nausea
   b. Diarrhea
   c. Fever
   d. Bladder pain

2. Both times that a urinalysis was done, the findings confirmed the presence of:
   a. Pus
   b. Bacteria
   c. Blood
   d. Protein

3. Lisa was referred to a physician who specialized in the treatment of:
   a. Female disorders
   b. Urinary tract disorders
   c. Colorectal disorders
   d. Endocrine disorders

4. The urologist performed which of the following procedures?
   a. Surgical removal of the bladder
   b. Surgical incision into the bladder
   c. Visual examination of the bladder
   d. Surgical fixation of the bladder

5. Which of the following abnormal findings were noted during the cystoscopy?
   a. Small cracks and sores that bleed
   b. Presence of cancerous lesions
   c. Presence of an infection
   d. A large bladder capacity

(text continues on page 160)

6. During the cystoscopy, the urologist also:
    a. Injected antibiotics into the bladder
    b. Used sterile salt water to stretch the bladder
    c. Applied medication to the bladder lining
    d. Cauterized the lesions to stop the bleeding

7. Which of the following statements is true about IC?
    a. It affects men more often than women
    b. It is a very common disorder
    c. The cause is clearly understood
    d. There is no known cure

8. Which of the following statements is true about IC?
    a. Each person with IC must learn by trial and error what makes symptoms better or worse
    b. All people with IC experience the same symptoms
    c. The same treatments are effective for everyone with IC
    d. The course of IC is predictable

9. Common symptoms of IC include:
    a. Urinary incontinence
    b. Fever
    c. Need to empty the bladder often
    d. Urinary retention

"The National Kidney Foundation is a terrific source of information."

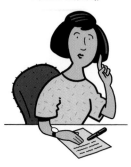

WEB SITES

National Kidney Foundation: www.kidney.org
American Urological Association: www.auanet.org
American Foundation for Urologic Disease: www.afud.org

PREFIX AND SUFFIX REVIEW

Tables 7-6 and 7-7 contain a review of selected prefixes and suffixes. Refer to these tables as necessary when you complete the exercises at the end of the chapter.

TABLE 7-6
PREFIX PRONUNCIATIONS AND MEANINGS

Prefix	Pronunciation Guide	Meaning
an-	ăn	without, absence of
anti-	ăn-tē	against
dys-	dĭs	painful, difficult
peri-	pĕr-ĭ	beside, near
poly-	pŏl-ē	many, much
retro-	rĕt-rō	behind, back

TABLE 7-7
SUFFIX PRONUNCIATIONS AND MEANINGS

Suffix	Pronunciation Guide	Meaning
-al, -ic -tic, -eal	ăl, ĭk tĭk, ē-ăl	pertaining to
-algia -dynia	ăl-jē-ă dĭn-ē-ă	pain
-dipsia	dĭp-sē-ă	thirst
-ectomy	ĕk-tō-mē	excision, surgical removal
-emia	ē-mē-ă	a condition of the blood
-genesis	jĕn-ĕ-sĭs	creating, producing
-gram	grăm	record
-iasis	ĭ-ă-sĭs	pathological condition or state
-itis	ī-tĭs	inflammation
-lith	lĭth	stone
-lysis	lĭ-sĭs	destruction of
-megaly	mĕg-ă-lē	enlargement
-meter	mĕ-tĕr	instrument for measuring
-pathy	pă-thē	disease
-pexy	pĕk-sē	surgical fixation
-scopy	skō-pē	visual examination
-stomy	stō-mē	mouth-like opening
-tome	tōm	cutting instrument
-tomy	tō-mē	cutting into, incision
-uria	ū-rē-ă	urine

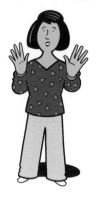

"Be sure to check your answers AFTER you've completed these exercises."

PRACTICE EXERCISES

Complete the following practice exercises. The answers can be found in Appendix G.

Matching

Match the following combining forms with the correct meanings. Some answers may be used more than once or not at all.

Exercise A

1. _____ py/o		a.	bacteria
2. _____ bacteri/o		b.	night
3. _____ cyst/o		c.	blood
4. _____ glyc/o		d.	pus
5. _____ olig/o		e.	renal pelvis
6. _____ hemat/o		f.	sugar
7. _____ lith/o		g.	deficient
8. _____ noct/o		h.	stone
9. _____ hem/o		i.	bladder

Exercise B

1. _____ pyel/o		a.	renal pelvis
2. _____ ureter/o		b.	peritoneum
3. _____ ren/o		c.	glomerulus
4. _____ ur/o		d.	bladder
5. _____ urethr/o		e.	stone

6. _____ nephr/o   f. kidney

7. _____ glomerulo   g. urethra

8. _____ peritone/o   h. urine

9. _____ urin/o   i. ureter

Word Building

*Using **only** the word parts in the lists provided, create medical terms with the indicated meanings.*

Prefixes	**Combining Forms**	**Suffixes**
an-	bacteri/o	-al
anti-	cyst/o	-algia
dys-	glomerul/o	-dynia
poly-	glyc/o	-ectomy
	hemat/o	-genesis
	lith/o	-gram
	nephr/o	-iasis
	noct/o	-ic
	olig/o	-itis
	py/o	-lith
	pyel/o	-lysis
	ren/o	-scopy
	ureter/o	-tic
	urethr/o	-uria
	ur/o	
	urin/o	

1. Absence of urine formation _____

2. Much urination _____

3. Pus in the urine _____

4. Painful or difficult urination _____

5. Pertaining to deficient urine (formation) _____

6. Pain in the urethra _____

7. Visual examination of the bladder _____

8. Blood in the urine _____

9. Condition of a kidney stone _____

10. Urination at night _____

11. Bacteria in the blood _____

12. Surgical removal of a ureter _____

13. Inflammation of the renal pelvis and kidney _____

14. A record of the urethra and bladder _____

15. Pertaining to urine _____

16. Producing sugar _____

17. Pertaining to the kidneys _____

18. Inflammation of the kidneys and glomerulus _____

19. Pertaining to against bacteria _____

20. Destruction of blood _____

Deciphering Terms

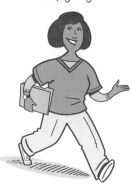

"You're doing great! keep going!"

Write the correct translation of the following medical terms.

1. renopathy _____

2. urethropexy _____

3. periurethral _____

4. cystectomy _____

5. nephrotomy _____

6. ureterostomy _____

7. glomerulonephritis _____

8. polydipsia _____

9. nephrectomy _____

10. nocturia _____

11. bacteriuria _____

12. hematuria _____

13. nephrolith _____

14. anuric _____

15. cystomegaly _____

16. retroperitoneal _____

True or False

Decide whether the following statements are true or false.

1. True   False   The term **enuresis** means involuntary urination during sleep.

2. True   False   The term **ureterodynia** means pain in the urethra.

3. True   False   The term **oliguric** means absence of urine formation.

4. True   False   The abbreviation **UTI** stands for urinary tract infection.

5. True   False   The combining form **vas/o** means void.

6. True   False   The term **diuresis** means deficient urine formation.

7. True   False   The abbreviation **ESRD** means end-stage renal disease.

8. True   False   The term **phimosis** refers to stenosis, or narrowing the foreskin opening.

9. True   False   **Interstitial cystitis** is a chronic condition of inflammation of the bladder lining.

10. True   False   The abbreviation **IVP** stands for intravenous pyelogram.

Fill in the Blank

Fill in the blanks below.

1. Two terms that mean *sugar in the urine* are

   _____ and _____.

2. An abbreviation that refers to *the final phase of kidney disease* is _____.

3. An abbreviation that refers to an *infection in the bladder* is

   _____.

4. The term that refers to *involuntary urination during sleep* is

   _____.

5. The term _____ means *stenosis, or narrowing of the foreskin opening.*

6. The term _____ refers to an *increased level of urea or protein waste in the blood.*

7. The term _____ refers to an *abnormal secretion of large amounts of urine.*

8. A *chronic condition of inflammation of the bladder lining* is

   _____.

9. The term _____ _____ refers to *pathologic changes in renal tissue that destroy nephrons and impair kidney function.*

10. The term _____ refers to *inflammation and infection caused by bacterial growth in the renal pelvis and kidney.*

11. When the bladder is full but the person is unable to urinate, the condition is known as _____

_____.

12. *Leakage of urine when one coughs or sneezes* is known as

_____ _____.

Common Diagnostic Tests

Write the definition of the following diagnostic tests.

1. **Blood urea nitrogen (BUN):**

2. **Culture and sensitivity (C&S):**

3. **24-hour urine specimen:**

4. **Intravenous pyelogram (IVP):**

5. **Serum creatinine:**

6. **Urinalysis (UA):**

"You're almost to the finish line. Don't stop now."

Multiple Choice Questions

Select the one best answer to the following multiple choice questions.

1. During her annual health check with her nurse practitioner, Mrs. Tran states that she has recently been experiencing involuntary leakage of urine when she laughs, coughs, or sneezes. Her symptoms are most consistent with which of the following disorders?

   a. Enuresis

   b. Polyuria

   c. Stress incontinence

   d. Nocturia

2. Mrs. Fernandez tells her physician that she has been having pain in her abdomen and lower pelvic area. To gather further information, the physician orders a KUB. This is an x-ray procedure that specifically looks at:

   a. Kidney, uterus, and bowel

   b. Kidney stones, urine, and blood

   c. Kyphosis, uremia, and bones

   d. Kidney, ureter, and bladder

3. Mr. Stadnick is a 73-year-old man who complains of increasing episodes of nocturia and frequency. Examination and testing reveal that he is not emptying his bladder completely when he urinates. The physician determines that he has a noncancerous enlargement of his prostate. Which of the following abbreviations is consistent with these findings?

   a. TURP

   b. BPH

   c. RP

   d. IVP

4. Ms. Johansen has had chronic complaints of frequency, urgency, dysuria, and intermittent low back and pelvic pain. She was initially treated with antibiotics for a presumed UTI, without any relief. A cystoscopy reveals that she has chronic inflammation of her bladder lining. This is most consistent with which of the following diagnoses?

   a. Urinary retention

   b. Interstitial cystitis

   c. Interstitial nephritis

   d. Uremia

5. Which of the following terms means *an instrument for measuring urine*?

   a. Urogram

   b. Urinoscopy

   c. Urinometer

   d. Urotome

You've completed chapter seven. Good for you!

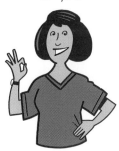

8

REPRODUCTIVE SYSTEM

The major function of both the male and female reproductive systems is procreation. These systems work together in a complementary fashion to join sperm and egg at the moment of conception to create a new human being.

STRUCTURE AND FUNCTION OF THE MALE REPRODUCTIVE SYSTEM

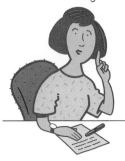

"Male sperm cells contain half of the genetic material needed to form a new human being."

Refer to Figure 8-1 as you read about the male reproductive system. **Sperm,** or **spermocytes** (sperm cells), are the male reproductive cells and carry half of the genetic material needed to form a new human being. They are produced in the **testicles,** or **testes,** and mature in the **epididymis.** The testes and epididymis are enclosed in a pouch called the **scrotum.** Mature sperm travel from the epididymis to the **vas deferens** and eventually to the **ejaculatory duct.** On ejaculation, sperm mixed in seminal fluid leave the body via the **urethra.**

In males, the urethra serves a dual purpose as a route for both urine and semen. The **seminal vesicles** and the **prostate gland** help ensure longer survival of the sperm by secreting an alkaline substance into the semen. The **bulbourethral glands** are located below the prostate; they add a sticky substance to the seminal fluid.

The penis is made up mostly of erectile tissue that becomes temporarily engorged with blood during sexual arousal. The distal end is known as the **glans penis** and is loosely covered by the **prepuce,** a fold of skin known as the foreskin. In some cases, it is

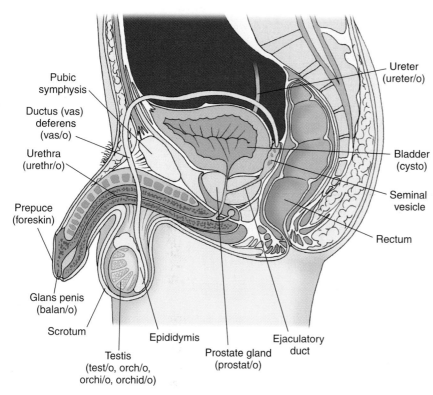

Pubic symphysis

Ductus (vas) deferens (vas/o)

Urethra (urethr/o)

Prepuce (foreskin)

Glans penis (balan/o)

Scrotum

Testis (test/o, orch/o, orchi/o, orchid/o)

Epididymis

Prostate gland (prostat/o)

Ejaculatory duct

Ureter (ureter/o)

Bladder (cysto)

Seminal vesicle

Rectum

Figure 8-1 The male reproductive system.

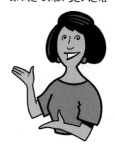

"In males, the urethra serves a dual purpose, as a route for both urine and semen."

partially or completely removed by the procedure known as *circumcision.*

STRUCTURE AND FUNCTION OF THE FEMALE REPRODUCTIVE SYSTEM

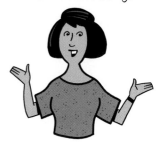

"An ovum contains the other half of the genetic material needed to form a new human being."

Refer to Figure 8-2 as you read about the female reproductive system. The ***ova,*** or ***oocytes*** (egg cells), are the female reproductive cells and carry the other half of the genetic material needed to form a new human being. They are produced in the ***ovaries;*** one ovum is released from alternating ovaries approximately every 28 days. The ovaries are two almond-shaped organs located on each side of the uterus. They serve two key functions: produce and house mature ova and release them in the process of ***ovulation*** each

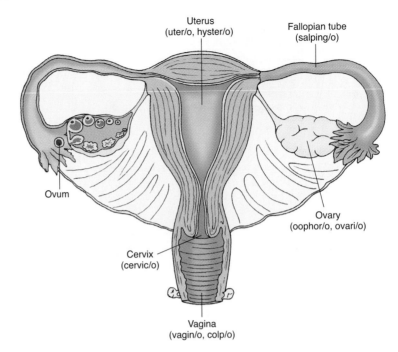

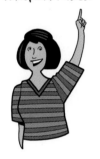

"The ovum is swept into the fallopian tube by the wavelike action of fingerlike projections on the fallopian tubes."

Figure 8-2   The female reproductive system.

month. The ovaries also release the sex hormones **progesterone** and **estrogen.**

After ovulation occurs, the ovum is swept into the **fallopian tubes** and makes its way to the **uterus.** If the ovum is fertilized, it begins to grow and is implanted into the uterine lining, which has thickened in preparation for potential implantation. If fertilization does not occur, the lining is shed in the process known as **menstruation.** The uterus is a hollow, thick-walled, muscular organ about the size and shape of a small inverted pear. When fertilization occurs, the uterus houses and protects the growing fetus until the time of birth. The inferior portion of the uterus, known as the **cervix,** projects into the superior end of the **vagina.** The vagina is a muscular tube that leads to the exterior. It is approximately 6 inches long and serves as the birth canal.

External female genitalia include the **vulva, clitoris, labia majora, labia minora,** and **Bartholin's glands.** The labia majora form the sides of the vulva. The smaller labia minora lie inside the labia majora. Bartholin's glands are mucus-secreting glands located on each side of and posterior to the vaginal opening. The clitoris is a small, sensitive erectile organ located at the anterior of the vulva. The mammary glands, or **breasts,** are milk-producing structures that become active after childbirth and supply nourishment for the newborn.

Memory Tip

The ovaries and the testes are somewhat round in shape, like the letter "o." Terms associated with the ovaries and testes usually have lots of o's in them: ovari/o, oophor/o, orch/o, orchi/o, orchid/o, and so on.

COMBINING FORMS

Tables 8-1 and 8-2 contain combining forms that pertain to the male and female reproductive systems along with examples of terms which utilize the combining form, and a pronunciation guide. Read out loud to yourself as you move from left to right across the table. Be sure to use the pronunciation guide so that you can learn to say the terms correctly.

TABLE 8-1

COMBINING FORMS RELATED TO THE REPRODUCTIVE SYSTEM

Combining Form	Meaning	Example	Meaning of New Term
balan/o	glans penis	balanitis (băl-ă-NĪ-tĭs)	inflammation of the glans penis
orch/o	testes	orchopathy (ŏr-KŌ-pă-thē)	disease of the testes
orchi/o		orchiectomy (ŏr-kē-ĔK-tō-mē)	surgical removal of the testes
orchid/o		orchidopexy (ŏr-kĭ-dō-PĔK-sē)	surgical fixation of the testes
test/o		testomegaly (tĕs-tō-MĔG-ă-lē)	enlargement of the testes
prostat/o	prostate	prostatoplasty (prŏs-tă-tō-PLĂS-tē)	surgical repair of the prostate
spermat/o	sperm	spermatogenesis (spĕr-măt-ō-JĔN-ĕ-sĭs)	producing sperm
sperm/o		aspermia (ă-SPĔR-mē-ă)	condition of no sperm
vas/o	vessel	vasotomy (văs-ŎT-ō-mē)	incision into a vessel

TABLE 8-2
OTHER COMBINING FORMS

Combining Form	Meaning	Example	Meaning of New Term
cervic/o	cervix	cervical (SĔR-vĭ-kăl)	pertaining to the cervix
colp/o	vagina	colposcopy (kŏl-PŎS-kō-pē)	visual examination of the vagina
vagin/o		vaginopexy (văj-ĭn-ō-PĔK-sē)	surgical fixation of the vagina
episi/o	vulva	episiotomy (ĕ-pĭs-ē-ŎT-ō-mē)	incision into the vulva (perineum)
vulv/o		vulvodynia (vŭl-vō-DĬN-ē-ă)	pain of the vulva
gynec/o	woman, female	gynecology (gī-nĕ-KŎL-ō-jē)	study of female (disorders)
hyster/o	uterus	hysterotomy (hĭs-tĕr-ŎT-ō-mē)	incision into the uterus
uter/o		uteral (Ū-tĕr-ăl)	pertaining to the uterus
lapar/o	abdomen	laparoscopy (lăp-ăr-ŎS-kō-pē)	visual examination of the abdomen
mamm/o	breast	mammoplasty (MĂM-ō-plăs-tē)	surgical repair of the breasts
mast/o		mastectomy (măs-TĔK-tō-mē)	surgical removal of the breasts
men/o	menses	dysmenorrhea (dĭs-mĕn-ō-RĒ-ă)	painful or difficult menstrual flow
nat/o	birth	natal (NĀ-tăl)	pertaining to birth
oophor/o	ovary	oophorectomy (ō-ŏf-ō-RĔK-tō-mē)	surgical removal of the ovaries
ovari/o		ovarioptosis (ō-vă-rē-ŏp-TŌ-sĭs)	prolapse of the ovary
salping/o	tubes (fallopian and eustachian)	salpingitis (săl-pĭn-JĪ-tĭs)	inflammation of the fallopian tubes

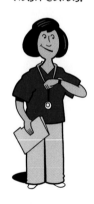

"Time to turn to your flash cards."

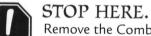

STOP HERE.
Remove the Combining Form Flash Cards for Chapter 8, and run through them at least 3 times before you continue.

PRACTICE EXERCISES

Use Table 8-1 to fill in the answers below.

1. _____ surgical removal of the testes

2. _____ incision into a vessel

3. _____ inflammation of the glans penis

4. _____ producing sperm

5. _____ surgical fixation of the testes

6. _____ enlargement of the testes

7. _____ disease of the testes

8. _____ surgical repair of the prostate

9. _____ condition of no sperm

10. Fill in the blanks with the appropriate anatomical term and/or combining form.

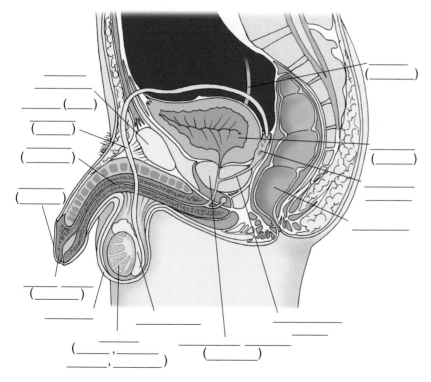

Figure 8-3

Use Table 8-2 to fill in the answers below.

11. _____ prolapse of the ovary

12. _____ pertaining to the cervix

13. _____ surgical removal of the ovaries

14. _____ pertaining to the uterus

15. _____ visual examination of the vagina

16. _____ surgical repair of the breasts

17. _____ painful or difficult menstrual flow

18. _____ incision into the vulva (perineum)

19. _____ pain of the vulva

20. _____ incision into the uterus

21. _____ visual examination of the abdomen

22. _____ inflammation of the fallopian tubes

23. _____ surgical removal of the breasts

24. _____ study of female (disorders)

25. _____ pertaining to birth

26. _____ surgical fixation of the vagina

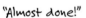

"Almost done!"

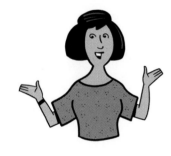

27. Fill in the blanks with the appropriate anatomical term and/or combining forms.

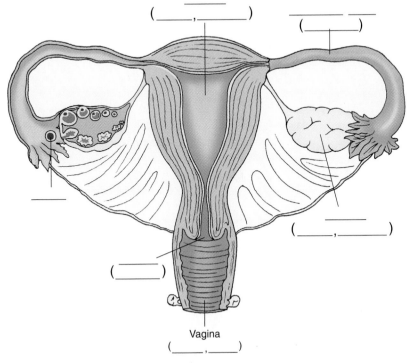

Vagina
(_____,_____)

Figure 8-4

ABBREVIATIONS

Table 8-3 lists some of the most common abbreviations related to the reproductive system as well as others often used in medical documentation.

TABLE 8-3

ABBREVIATIONS

Female Reproductive System

C-section	cesarean section
D&C	dilation and curettage
GYN	gynecology

(continues on page 178)

Female Reproductive System

IUD	intrauterine device
IVF	in vitro fertilization
LMP	last menstrual period
OB-GYN	obstetrics and gynecology
OC	oral contraceptive
Pap	Papanicolaou's smear
PID	pelvic inflammatory disease
TAH	total abdominal hysterectomy
TAH-BSO	total abdominal hysterectomy, bilateral salpingo-oophorectomy
♀	symbol for female

Male Reproductive System

BPH	benign prostatic hypertrophy; also called benign prostatic hyperplasia (Fig. 8-5)

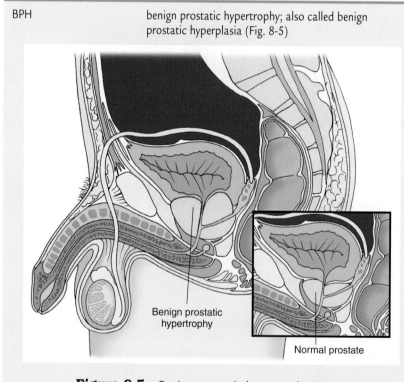

Benign prostatic hypertrophy

Normal prostate

Figure 8-5   Benign prostatic hypertrophy (BPH).

Male Reproductive System

TURP	transurethral resection of the prostate
♂	symbol for male

Male and Female Reproductive Systems

GU	genitourinary
STD	sexually transmitted disease
VD	venereal disease

 STOP HERE.
Remove the Abbreviation Flash Cards for Chapter 8, and run through them at least 3 times before you continue.

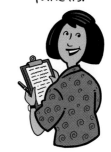

"The symbols ♂ and ♀ are commonly used in charting to refer to male and female patients."

PATHOLOGY TERMS

Table 8-4 includes terms that relate to diseases or abnormalities of the reproductive system. Use the pronunciation guide, and say the terms out loud as you read them. This will help you get in the habit of saying them properly.

TABLE 8-4
PATHOLOGY TERMS

Female Reproductive System

candidiasis (kăn-dĭ-DĪ-ă-sĭs)	vaginal fungal infection caused by *Candida albicans*; key Sx include itching; burning; thick, curdy discharge
ectopic pregnancy (ĕk-TŎ-pĭk)	fertilized ovum is implanted outside of the uterus, often in the fallopian tube (also called tubal pregnancy [Fig. 8-6]
endometriosis (ĕn-dō-mē-trē-Ō-sĭs)	endometrial tissue grows in abnormal sites in lower abdominopelvic area; causes severe dysmenorrhea (Fig. 8-7)
fibroids (FĪ-broyds)	benign uterine tumors
uterine prolapse (PRŌ-lăps)	protrusion of uterus through the vaginal opening

Male Reproductive System

benign prostatic hypertrophy (BPH) (bē-NĪN prŏs-TĂT-ĭc hī-PĔR-trŏ-fē)	noncancerous enlargement of the prostate gland; common in elderly men (see Fig. 8-5)

(continues on page 180)

179

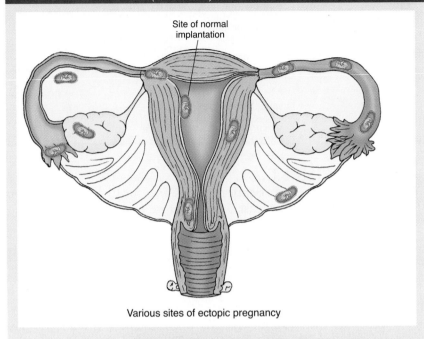

Site of normal
implantation

Various sites of ectopic pregnancy

Figure 8-6 Ectopic pregnancy.

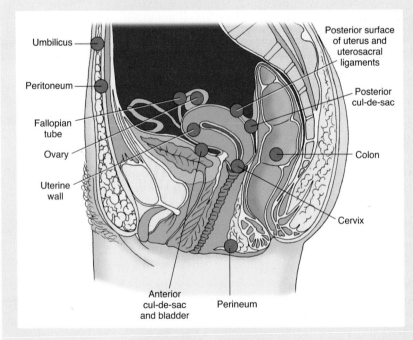

Umbilicus

Peritoneum

Fallopian
tube

Ovary

Uterine
wall

Anterior
cul-de-sac
and bladder

Posterior surface
of uterus and
uterosacral
ligaments

Posterior
cul-de-sac

Colon

Cervix

Perineum

Figure 8-7 Endometriosis.

Male Reproductive System

cryptorchidism (krĭpt-ŎR-kĭd-ĭsm)	failure of one or both testes to descend into the scrotum
impotence (ĬM-pŏ-tĕns)	inability of a male to achieve or maintain an erection

Male and Female Reproductive Systems

chlamydia (klă-MĬD-ē-ă)	the most common STD, a bacterial vaginal infection caused by *Chlamydia trachomatis*
genital warts	STD, caused by human papillomavirus; causes painless cauliflower-like warts; a cause of cervical cancer in women
gonorrhea (gŏn-ō-RĒ-ă)	STD, caused by *Neisseria gonorrhoeae*; causes inflammation of mucous membranes
herpes genitalis (HĔRP-ēs jĕn-ĭ-TĂL-ĭs)	STD, caused by herpes simplex virus type 2; causes painful vesicles (Fig. 8-8)

A 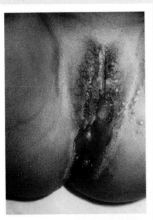 B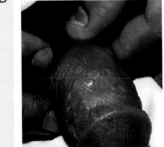

Figure 8-8 Herpes genitalis as manifested in female (A) and male (B) patients. (From Dillon PM: Nursing Health Assessment. Philadelphia, FA Davis, pp 543 and 577.)

sterility (stĕr-ĬL-ĭ-tē)	inability to produce offspring
syphilis (SĬF-ĭ-lĭs)	STD, key Sx include skin lesions; eventually fatal unless treated
trichomoniasis (trĭk-ō-mō-NĪ-ă-sĭs)	STD, infestation with parasite genus *Trichomonas*; key Sx include vaginitis, urethritis, and cystitis

 STOP HERE.
Remove the Pathology Terms Flash Cards for Chapter 8, and run through them at least 3 times before you continue.

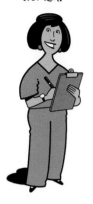

"The Papanicolaou smear is often called the Pap smear and is a critical test for women."

COMMON DIAGNOSTIC TESTS

Cryosurgery: destruction of abnormal tissue by freezing

Dilation and curettage (D&C): cervix is dilated, and endometrial lining of uterus is scraped

Needle biopsy: tissue or fluid is drawn through a large-gauge needle for analysis

Papanicolaou's smear: cells are removed from the cervix and studied for cancer or other abnormalities

Pelvic sonography: ultrasound imaging of structures in female pelvis

Prostate-specific antigen (PSA): blood test used to screen for prostate cancer

Transurethral resection of the prostate (TURP): removal of tissue from the prostate gland with an endoscope via the urethra

Tubal ligation: sterilization procedure in which fallopian tubes are cut and ligated (Fig. 8-9)

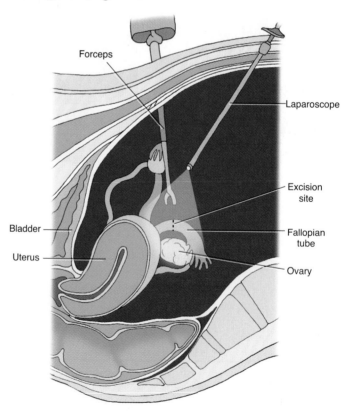

Figure 8-9 Tubal ligation.

Vasectomy: sterilization procedure in which a small section of the vas deferens is removed (Fig. 8-10)

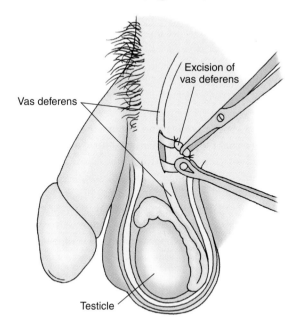

Figure 8-10   Vasectomy.

CASE STUDY

Read the following case study, and answer the questions that follow. Most of the terms are included in this chapter. Refer to the Glossary or to your medical dictionary for the other terms.

Endometriosis

Susan Brownlee is a 32-year-old woman with a history of dysmenorrhea since the age of 13. Her primary symptoms include pelvic pain and cramping prior to and during her menses. Severity of Sx caused her to occasionally miss 1 to 2 days of school each month when she was young. Over time, her symptoms have slowly worsened, currently causing her to miss an average of 2 to 3 days of work each month. Treatment with acetaminophen and NSAIDs provided only partial relief, so she was eventually started on hormonal therapy.

Susan has been married for 8 years and has been trying to get pregnant for the past 5 years. During evaluation and treatment for infertility, a laparoscopy was performed, and a diagnosis of endometriosis was confirmed. Surgical treatment was performed at the same time, in which endometrial implants and

(continues on page 184)

cysts were removed from the outer surface of her ovaries and fallopian tubes. She was informed that this procedure may reduce her dysmenorrhea symptoms and increase the chance of a successful pregnancy but that the only definitive treatment for endometriosis is a total hysterosalpingo-oophorectomy. Susan states that she understands this but wants to postpone that decision because of her wish to have children.

Endometriosis occurs in 10% to 15% of all women of reproductive age and in 50% of infertile women. The cause is not clearly understood, but there seems to be a genetic predisposition. One theory involves the implantation of endometrial cells from menstrual flow, which moves up the fallopian tubes and into the pelvic cavity. Another theory involves the spread of endometrial cells through blood and lymph vessels. Other theories list possible immunological factors. A presumptive diagnosis is made based on history and symptoms, but a definitive diagnosis is made by the performance of a laparoscopy, which allows direct visualization of the reproductive organs and surrounding structures. Treatment depends on the severity of the symptoms. Options include analgesics, hormone therapy, and surgery.

Case Study Questions

1. Since the age of 13, Susan has experienced:
    a. Painful or difficult menstrual flow
    b. Absence of menses
    c. Excessive menstrual flow
    d. Fear of menses

2. Treatment for her dysmenorrhea has included:
    a. Cystoscopy with bladder distention
    b. Steroids
    c. Nonsteroidal anti-inflammatory drugs
    d. Hysterectomy

3. The diagnosis of endometriosis was confirmed by:
    a. Visual examination of the bladder
    b. Incision into the abdomen
    c. Visual examination of the abdomen
    d. Visual examination of the vagina and cervix

4. What was removed from Susan's abdomen during her laparoscopy?
    a. Her uterus
    b. Her fallopian tubes
    c. Cancerous growths
    d. Endometrial tissue

5. As a result of the surgical procedure, Susan understands that:
   a. Her endometriosis is probably cured
   b. Her symptoms of dysmenorrhea will likely worsen
   c. Her chances of becoming pregnant have increased
   d. The only reliable cure for her endometriosis is surgical removal of her fallopian tubes

6. Which of the following statements is true regarding endometriosis?
   a. It is common among women
   b. There is no relationship to infertility
   c. Severity of symptoms tends to remain constant over time
   d. Endometrial tissue proliferates in abnormal areas

7. Which of the following statements is true regarding endometriosis?
   a. The most effective permanent treatment is complete removal of uterus, fallopian tubes, and ovaries
   b. A definite diagnosis can be made based on history and current symptoms
   c. Standard treatment for endometriosis involves the use of steroids
   d. Symptoms tend to improve as the woman ages

WEB SITES

American Society for Reproductive Medicine: www.asrm.org
Endometriosis Association: www.endometriosisassn.org
North American Menopause Society: www.menopause.org

PREFIX AND SUFFIX REVIEW

Tables 8-5 and 8-6 contain a review of selected prefixes and suffixes. Refer to these tables as necessary when you complete the exercises at the end of the chapter.

TABLE 8-5
PREFIX PRONUNCIATIONS AND MEANINGS

Prefix	Pronunciation Guide	Meaning
a-, an-	ā, ăn	without, absence of
circum-	sĕr-kŭm	around
dys-	dĭs	painful, difficult
hyper-	hī-pĕr	excessive, above
multi-	mŭl-tē	many, much
neo-	nē-ō	new
oligo-	ōl-ĭ-gō	deficient
peri-	pĕr-ĭ	near, surrounding
post-	pōst	after, following
pre-	prē	before, forward
retro-	rĕt-rō	behind, back

TABLE 8-6
SUFFIX PRONUNCIATIONS AND MEANINGS

Suffix	Pronunciation Guide	Meaning
-al, -ia, -tic	ăl, ē-ă, tĭc	pertaining to
-algia -dynia	ăl-jē-ă dĭn-ē-ă	pain
-cele	sēl	hernia
-ectasis	ĕk-tă-sĭs	dilation, expansion
-ectomy	ĕk-tō-mē	excision, surgical removal
-esthesia	ĕs-thē-zē-ă	sensation
-gram	grăm	record
-graphy	gră-fē	process of recording
-gravida	grăv-ĭ-dă	pregnant woman
-ia, -ism	ē-ă, ĭzm	condition
-itis	ī-tĭs	inflammation
-logist	lō-jĭst	specialist in the study of
-logy	lō-jē	study of
-oma	ō-mă	tumor

Suffix	Pronunciation Guide	Meaning
-pause	pawz	cessation
-pexy	pĕk-sē	surgical fixation
-plasm -plasia	plăzm pla-zē-ă	formation, growth
-plasty	plăs-tē	surgical repair
-rrhaphy	ră-fē	suture, suturing
-rrhea	rē-ă	flow, discharge
-rrhexis	rĕk-sĭs	rupture
-scope	skōp	instrument to view
-scopy	skō-pē	visual examination
-stenosis	stĕ-nō-sĭs	narrowing, stricture
-tomy	tō-mē	cutting into, incision

PRACTICE EXERCISES

Complete the following practice exercises. The answers can be found in Appendix G.

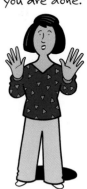

"To get the most out of these exercises, be sure to check your answers only AFTER you are done."

Matching

Match the following combining forms with the correct meanings. Some answers may be used more than once or not at all.

Exercise A

1. _____ orch/o

2. _____ balan/o

3. _____ vas/o

4. _____ spermat/o

5. _____ orchi/o

6. _____ prostat/o

7. _____ orchid/o

a. female

b. vulva

c. testes

d. neck

e. tube

f. ovary

g. glans penis

8. _____ oophor/o   h. sperm

9. _____ test/o   i. prostate

10. _____ ovari/o   j. vessel

11. _____ gynec/o   k. birth

12. _____ nat/o   l. uterus

13. _____ sperm/o

Exercise B

1. _____ salping/o   a. abdomen

2. _____ men/o   b. cervix

3. _____ cervic/o   c. sperm

4. _____ lapar/o   d. prostate

5. _____ hyster/o   e. tube

6. _____ mast/o   f. uterus

7. _____ colp/o   g. menses

8. _____ vagin/o   h. breast

9. _____ uter/o   i. testes

10. _____ mamm/o   j. vagina

11. _____ episi/o   k. vulva

12. _____ vulv/o   l. vessel

Word Building

*Using **only** the word parts in the lists provided, create medical terms with the indicated meanings.*

Prefixes	Combining Forms	Suffixes
a-	balan/o	-al
an-	cervic/o	-algia
dys-	colp/o	-cele

multi-	episi/o	-dynia
neo-	gynec/o	-ectomy
oligo-	hyster/o	-esthesia
peri-	lapar/o	-gram
retro-	mamm/o	-gravida
	mast/o	-ia
	men/o	-ism
	nat/o	-itis
	oophor/o	-logist
	orchid/o	-oma
	prostat/o	-pause
	salping/o	-pexy
	sperm/o	-plasia
	vagin/o	-plasm
	vas/o	-rrhaphy
		-rrhexis
		-scope
		-stenosis
		-tomy

"You're off to a great start. Keep up the good work."

1. inflammation of the glans penis _____

2. incision into the vulva (perineum) _____

3. a condition of absent testes _____

4. surgical fixation of the testes _____

5. a condition of deficient sperm _____

6. pertaining to near (the time of)
   birth _____

7. painful or difficult formation or
   growth _____

8. new formation or growth _____

9. pertaining to behind the vagina _____

10. absence of sensation _____

11. narrowing of a vessel _____

12. painful prostate _____

13. inflammation of the cervix _____

14. suturing of the vagina _____

15. specialist in the study of female
    (disorders) _____

16. instrument used to view the
    abdomen _____

17. surgical removal of the uterus _____

18. record (x-ray) of a breast _____

19. surgical fixation of a breast _____

20. cessation of menses _____

21. many pregnancies _____

22. tumor of the ovary _____

23. herniation of the vagina _____

24. rupture of a (fallopian) tube _____

Deciphering Terms

Write the correct translation of the following medical terms.

1. The abbreviation Gyn stands for _____

2. Fibroids are _____

3. OC stands for _____

4. Ectopic pregnancy occurs when _____

   _____

5. The abbreviation TURP stands for _____

6. Endometriosis occurs when _____

   _____

7. TAH-BSO stands for _____

8. Trichomoniasis is _____

9. orchiectasis _____

10. salpingo-oophorectomy _____

11. balanoplasty _____

12. dysplasia _____

13. neoplastic _____

14. mammography _____

15. laparoscopy _____

16. orchidorrhaphy _____

17. multigravida _____

18. menopause _____

19. hyperplasia _____

20. prostatocele _____

True or False

Decide whether the following statements are true or false.

1. True   False   **Herpes genitalis** is caused by herpes simplex virus type 2.

2. True   False   The abbreviation **PID** stands for pelvic invasive disorder.

3. True   False   The key symptoms of **candidiasis** are itching, burning and a thick curdy discharge.

"You're making great progress! Keep going!"

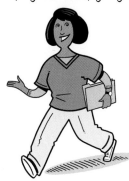

4. True   False   The abbreviation **IUD** stands for inter-urinary disorder.

5. True   False   **Uterine prolapse** is a herniation of the vaginal wall.

6. True   False   **VD** and **STD** are the same thing.

7. True   False   The symbol for male is ♂

8. True   False   The symbol for female is ♀

9. True   False   The abbreviation **GU** stands for gonorrhea.

10. True   False   **Cryptorchidism** is the absence of testes.

11. True   False   The abbreviation **LMP** stands for last menstrual period.

12. True   False   The abbreviation **D&C** stands for a type of contraceptive.

13. True   False   **Genital warts** are caused by the human papilloma virus.

14. True   False   **BPH** and **TAH** are the same thing.

15. True   False   **Chlamydia** is the most common STD in the U.S.

Fill in the Blank

Fill in the blanks below.

1. When a fertilized ovum is implanted outside of the uterus, it is called a(n) _____ pregnancy.

2. Lacey has dysmenorrhea due to endometrial tissue growth in her abdominopelvic area. This condition is known as _____.

3. _____ is an STD which is eventually fatal
   if not treated.

4. Olga is a 54-year-old woman who underwent a _____
   _____ _____, abbreviated TAH, due to
   noncancerous uterine tumors also known as
   _____.

5. Marcella will see her OB-GYN physician every week
   during her 9th month of pregnancy. OB-GYN stands
   for _____ _____ _____.

6. _____ is an STD caused by a parasite.

7. Danielle is using OC as her method of birth control. OC
   stands for _____ _____.

8. Danielle's nurse practitioner recommends that she have a
   Pap test once a year. *Pap* is an abbreviation that stands for
   _____ _____.

9. _____ is the inability to produce offspring.

10. Carla and her husband have tried unsuccessfully for 4 years
    to have a baby. They are now considering IVF, which is
    _____ _____ _____.

11. The abbreviation *TAH-BSO* stands for _____ _____
    _____, _____ _____.

12. Nicholas is a 65-year-old man with *BPH*, or _____ _____
    _____.

13. Nicholas will undergo a procedure known as a *TURP*, or
    _____ _____ _____ _____ _____.

14. The inability of the man to achieve or maintain erection is
    known as _____.

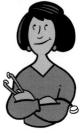

"You learn by repetition, so keep going!"

COMMON DIAGNOSTIC TESTS

Write the definition of the following diagnostic tests.

1. **Cryosurgery:**

2. **Dilation and curettage (D&C):**

3. **Needle biopsy:**

4. **Papanicolaou's smear:**

5. **Pelvic sonography:**

6. **Prostate-specific antigen (PSA):**

7. **Transurethral resection of the prostate (TURP):**

8. **Tubal ligation:**

9. **Vasectomy:**

Multiple Choice Questions

Select the one best answer to the following multiple choice questions.

1. Ms. Andretti came to the clinic today complaining of severe menstrual pain and cramping. Which of the following medical terms best describes her complaint?

   a. Menitis

   b. Vaginorrhea

   c. Dysmenorrhea

   d. Cervicitis

2. Mrs. Ramirez had a painful ovarian cyst on her left side. The ovary and the cyst were surgically removed through her lower abdomen with a small endoscope. The proper name for this procedure is a:

   a. Laparoscopic oophorectomy

   b. Colposcopic oophorotomy

   c. Vaginoscopic salpingo-oophorectomy

   d. Laparoscopic hysterectomy

3. Mr. Smyth had to be circumcised due to chronic balanitis. He had:

   a. A continual prostate infection

   b. Constant inflammation of his testes

   c. Constant inflammation of his glans penis

   d. Continual pain of his vas deferens

4. Mrs. Brown is 6 months pregnant and sees her physician each month for care. This type of care is known as:

   a. Prenatal care

   b. Perinatal care

   c. Postnatal care

   d. Circumnatal care

"You've completed the entire chapter. What a great accomplishment!"

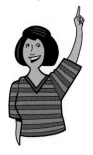

5. Which of the following combining forms does **not** mean testes?

    a.   test/o

    b.   orchi/o

    c.   orchid/o

    d.   oophor/o

ENDOCRINE SYSTEM

9

STRUCTURE AND FUNCTION

The endocrine system regulates the hormones in the body. Various organs of the endocrine system produce and secrete these hormones in order to maintain homeostasis (Fig. 9-1). The **pituitary gland,** often called the "master gland," is a small structure located in the brain. It has this nickname because it controls all the other glands in the body. It produces many hormones, including **growth hormone (GH),** which promotes growth of body structures; **thyroid-stimulating hormone (TSH),** which affects the thyroid; various hormones that affect sexual development and functioning; and hormones that help to regulate fluid volume and blood pressure.

The **thyroid gland** is located in the neck inferior to the larynx and anterior to the trachea. It produces the thyroid hormones **(T3 and T4),** important in the regulation of metabolism, and **calcitonin,** which helps to regulate calcium levels. The **parathyroid glands** lie on the surface of the thyroid gland. They produce **parathyroid hormone (PTH),** which works with calcitonin to regulate calcium content in the bones and the blood. The **adrenal glands** sit on top of the two kidneys. They secrete **aldosterone,** which is responsible for water and electrolyte balance. They also produce **cortisol,** the body's natural steroid, and **epinephrine** (also known as *adrenalin*), which is responsible for the "fight or flight" survival response (see table next page).

The **pancreas** lies in the upper left quadrant of the abdomen and plays an active role in the digestive system as well as the endocrine system. It secretes the hormones **insulin** and **glucagon.** Insulin is responsible for the storage and use of carbohydrates and decreases blood glucose levels. Glucagon increases blood glucose levels. These two hormones work together to maintain an optimal

"The tiny pituitary gland has been nicknamed the 'master gland' because it controls all other glands in the body."

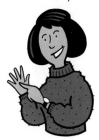

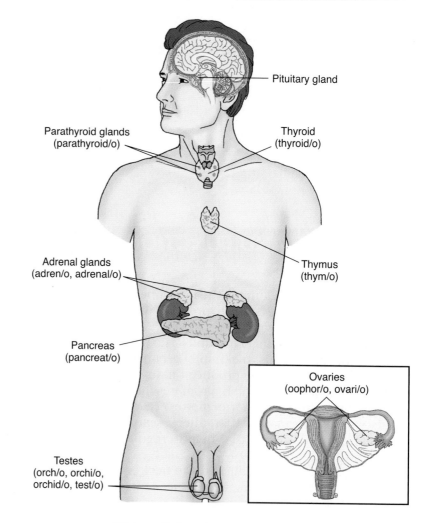

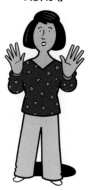

"If you feel threatened or frightened, your adrenal glands give you a dose of epinephrine, which prepares you for action."

Figure 9-1   The endocrine system.

THE FIGHT OR FLIGHT RESPONSE

This response is also known as the *"fright, fight, or flight response"* and stimulates the adrenal glands to secrete cortisol and epinephrine (adrenalin). This is a survival response that prepares the body for action. These hormones have the following effect on the body:

↑ **heart rate**
↑ **blood pressure**
↑ **blood glucose**
↑ **respiratory rate**

level of blood glucose to ensure that the body's energy needs are met. However, when dysregulation occurs, as with **diabetes mellitus,** blood glucose levels may go too high (hyperglycemia) or too low (hypoglycemia).

The tiny **pineal gland** produces the hormone **melatonin,** which helps to regulate the sleep-wake cycle. The **thymus** secretes its own hormones and plays an active role in the immune system in the very young but becomes less active upon aging.

Hormones often work in pairs to achieve the goal of homeostasis. For example, the thyroid gland produces calcitonin, which helps bones absorb calcium to keep them dense and strong. In this process, calcium is taken from the blood, lowering the blood calcium level. However, if blood calcium levels drop too low (hypocalcemia), the parathyroid glands respond by secreting PTH, which causes calcium to leave the bones and reenter the blood, thus raising calcium levels back to normal.

Another example of hormone teamwork is insulin and glucagon, which work together to regulate blood glucose levels. These hormones generally work well together, but when they do not the cause may be a disease known as diabetes mellitus (DM). The classic signs of new onset or undiagnosed diabetes are the three "polys": **polydipsia** (much thirst); **polyphagia** (much eating), which indicates an increased appetite; and **polyuria** (much urination). In spite of eating more, the person may lose weight because of faulty carbohydrate metabolism; in spite of drinking more, the person may become dehydrated due to polyuria. In severe cases, as these symptoms worsen and blood glucose levels rise, lethargy may progress to loss of consciousness. This is called **diabetic ketoacidosis (DKA),** otherwise known as a diabetic coma. Treatment includes admission to the hospital for fluid resuscitation (rehydration) and insulin therapy.

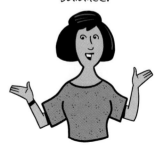

"Hormones work in pairs to achieve a healthy balance."

COMBINING FORMS

Table 9-1 contains combining forms that pertain to the endocrine system, examples of terms that utilize the combining form, and a pronunciation guide. Notice that some terms from the reproductive system are repeated here. This is because some reproductive organs (ovaries and testes) play an active role in the endocrine system. Read out loud to yourself as you move from left to right across the table. Be sure to use the pronunciation guide so that you learn to say the terms correctly.

TABLE 9-1
COMBINING FORMS RELATED TO THE ENDOCRINE SYSTEM

Combining Form	Meaning	Example	Meaning of New Term
aden/o	gland	adenopathy (ăd-ĕ-NŎP-ă-thē)	disease of a gland
adrenal/o adren/o	adrenal gland	adrenalectomy (ăd-rē-năl-ĔK-tō-mē) adrenal (ăd-rē-năl)	surgical removal of the adrenal gland pertaining to the adrenal gland
calc/o	calcium	hypercalcemia (hī-pĕr-kăl-SĒ-mē-ă)	excessive calcium in the blood
gluc/o glyc/o	sugar, glucose	glucogenesis (gloo-kō-JĔN-ĕ-sĭs) glycosuria (glĭ-kō-SŪ-rē-ă)	creating glucose sugar in the urine
hydr/o	water	hydrolysis (hī-DRŎL-ĭ-sĭs)	destruction of water
oophor/o ovari/o	ovary	oophorectomy (ō-ŏf-ō-RĔK-tō-mē) ovarioptosis (ō-vă-rē-ŏp-TŌ-sĭs)	surgical removal of the ovaries prolapse of the ovary
orch/o orchi/o orchid/o test/o	testes	orchopathy (ŏr-KŎ-pă-thē) orchiectomy (ŏr-kē-ĔK-tō-mē) orchidopexy (ŏr-kĭ-dō-PĔK-sē) testomegaly (tĕs-tō-MĔG-ă-lē)	disease of the testes surgical removal of the testes surgical fixation of the testes enlargement of the testes
pancreat/o	pancreas	pancreatography (păn-krē-ă-TŎG-ră-fē)	process of recording the pancreas
parathyroid/o	parathyroid	parathyroidectomy (păr-ă-thī-royd-ĔK-tō-mē)	surgical removal of the parathyroid gland
thym/o	thymus	thymoma (thī-MŌ-mă)	tumor of the thymus
thyroid/o	thyroid	thyroiditis (thī-royd-Ī-tĭs)	inflammation of the thyroid
toxic/o	toxin, poison	toxicologist (tŏks-ĭ-KŎL-ō-jĭst)	specialist in the study of toxins

hyperglucemia

STOP HERE.
Remove the Combining Forms Flash Cards for Chapter 9, and run through them at least 3 times before you continue.

PRACTICE EXERCISE

Use Table 9-1 to fill in the answers below.

1. _____ enlargement of the testes

2. _____ surgical removal of the parathyroid gland

3. _____ surgical fixation of the testes

4. _____ surgical removal of the adrenal gland

5. _____ disease of a gland

6. _____ specialist in the study of toxins

7. _____ excessive calcium in the blood

8. _____ disease of the testes

9. _____ creating glucose

10. _____ destruction of water

11. _____ tumor of the thymus

12. _____ surgical removal of the ovaries

13. _____ sugar in the urine

14. _____ pertaining to the adrenal gland

15. _____ surgical removal of the testes

16. _____ inflammation of the thyroid

17. _____ prolapse of the ovary

18. _____ process of recording the pancreas

19. Fill in the blanks with the appropriate anatomical term and/or combining form.

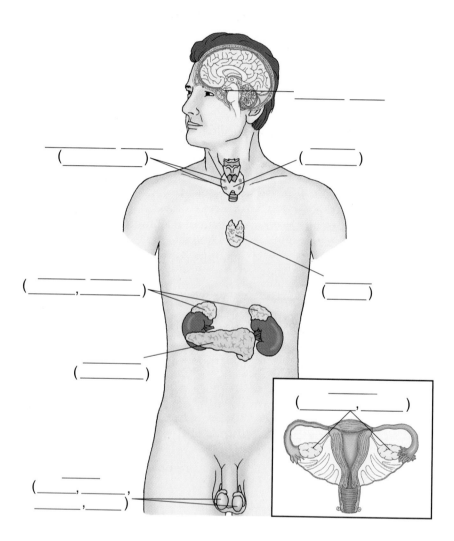

Figure 9-2

ABBREVIATIONS

Table 9-2 lists some of the most common abbreviations related to the endocrine system as well as others often used in medical documentation.

A common area of confusion is the finger stick blood sugar (fsbs) and the fasting blood sugar (FBS). Please note the following differences.

FBS: The person has fasted (not eaten anything) for a designated time, usually 8 to 12 hours. The blood is drawn from a vein with a needle and syringe or with a device called a vacutainer (needle attached to a vacuum-sealed tube). The blood specimen is tested in the laboratory.

fsbs: Blood sugar may be checked at any time but is usually checked just prior to meals. A drop of capillary blood is obtained by poking the tip of the finger with a lancet (tiny sharp blade). The blood is tested immediately using an instrument called a glucometer.

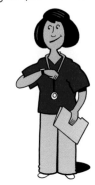

The FBS requires an 8-12 hour fast. The fsbs is often checked just prior to meals.

TABLE 9-2	
ABBREVIATIONS	
ADH	antidiuretic hormone
BS	blood sugar (also known as blood glucose [BG])
Ca	calcium
CA	cancer
DM	diabetes mellitus
FBS	fasting blood sugar
fsbs	finger stick blood sugar
GH	growth hormone
IDDM	insulin-dependent diabetes mellitus (type I diabetes)
K	potassium
Na	sodium
NIDDM	noninsulin-dependent diabetes mellitus (type II diabetes)
PTH	parathyroid hormone
T3, T4	thyroid hormones
TSH	thyroid-stimulating hormone

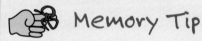

Memory Tip

The following terms are easier to understand and remember when you notice that they include the chemistry abbreviations for each of the electrolytes.

		↑ level	↓ level
potassium:	K	hyper_k_alemia	hypo_k_alemia
sodium:	Na	hyper_na_tremia	hypo_na_tremia
calcium:	Ca	hyper_ca_lcemia	hypo_ca_lcemia

Also remember: hyper- means *excessive or above normal*
hypo- means *below normal*
-emia means *blood*

STOP HERE.

Remove the Abbreviation Flash Cards for Chapter 9, and run through them at least 3 times before you continue.

PATHOLOGY TERMS

Table 9-3 includes terms that relate to diseases or abnormalities of the endocrine system. Use the pronunciation guide, and say the terms out loud as you read them. This will help you get in the habit of saying them properly.

TABLE 9-3	
PATHOLOGY TERMS	
Addison's disease	disorder in which adrenal cortex is destroyed, resulting in chronic metabolic disorder that requires hormone replacement therapy
cretinism (KRĒ-tĭn-ĭzm)	arrested physical and mental development caused by insufficient thyroid secretion in infancy (Fig. 9-3)
Cushing's (KOOSH-ĭngs) **syndrome**	disorder caused by hypersecretion of glucocorticoids by the adrenal gland, resulting in altered fat distribution and muscle weakness

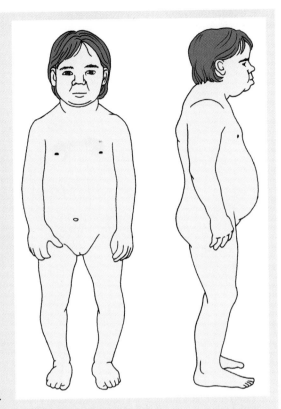

Figure 9-3 Cretinism.

diabetes (dī-ă-BĒ-tēz) **mellitus** (mĕl-Ī-tĭs) **(DM)**	chronic metabolic disorder in which the pancreas secretes insufficient amounts of insulin or the body is insulin-resistant
dwarfism	hyposecretion of growth hormone during childhood, resulting in an abnormally small adult (Fig. 9-4)
exophthalmos (ĕks-ŏf-THĂL-mōs)	abnormal protrusion of the eyeballs (Fig. 9-5)
gigantism	hypersecretion of growth hormone during childhood, resulting in an abnormally large adult (see Fig. 9-4)
Graves' disease	hyperthyroidism caused by an autoimmune response; may cause exophthalmos
myxedema mĭks-ĕ-DĒ-mă	nonpitting edema in connective tissue caused by advanced hypothyroidism
retinopathy (rĕt-ĭn-ŎP-ă-thē)	disease of the retina, often caused by diabetes

(continues on page 206)

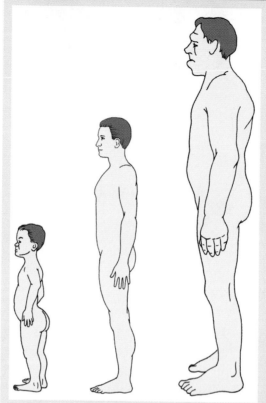

Figure 9-4 Dwarfism and gigantism.

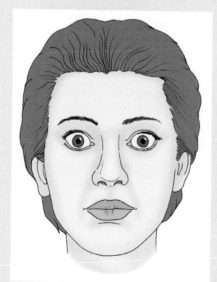

Figure 9-5 Exophthalmos.

STOP HERE.
Remove the Pathology Term Flash Cards for Chapter 9, and
run through them at least 3 times before you continue.

COMMON DIAGNOSTIC TESTS

Fasting blood glucose (FBG): also called FBS; tests blood glucose
levels after a fast for 8 to 12 hours; used to screen for diabetes

finger stick blood sugar (fsbs): also called finger stick blood
glucose (FSBG); blood glucose tested from a drop of capillary blood
obtained by pricking the finger

Glucose tolerance test (GTT): measures blood glucose levels at
specified intervals after ingestion of glucose

Glycosylated hemoglobin (Hgb A1c): reflects the average blood
glucose level over the past 3 to 4 months

Thyroid-stimulating hormone: reflects thyroid function; tested
to detect hypothyroidism

CASE STUDY

*Read the following case study, and answer the questions that follow. Most of
the terms are included in this chapter. Refer to the Glossary or to your medical
dictionary for the other terms.*

Diabetes

*Marsha Bloom is a 43-year-old female with a history of good health other than
mild obesity. She reports a recent 25-pound weight loss over 3 months without
dieting. She describes an increased appetite and states that she has been eating
more than usual. She has also had polydipsia, polyphagia, and polyuria. Marsha
complains of increasing fatigue in spite of getting 8 to 9 hours of sleep each
night. Her greatest concern is a recent realization that her vision has worsened
significantly. She describes being unable to recognize her friend at the grocery
store until she was just a few feet away from her. This is what prompted her to
seek medical attention.*

*Results of a GTT indicate a rise in blood glucose to more than 300 and confirm
a diagnosis of type II diabetes. Marsha was started on oral agents to control her
blood glucose levels and was referred to a diabetic educator to learn more about
her disease and to develop a plan for management.*

*Three months later, after meeting with the diabetic educator and being
evaluated by her ophthalmologist, Marsha began a regular exercise program and
made some positive changes in her diet. Over the past 3 months, she has lost
another 20 pounds, has noted an improvement in her vision, and commented that
her "poly" symptoms have resolved. Best of all, she states that her energy level has
increased dramatically.*

"Here's a great
case to study.
You'll undoubtedly
care for many
diabetic patients."

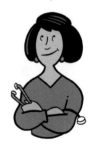

(continues on page 208)

Noninsulin-dependent diabetes mellitus (NIDDM), also known as **type II diabetes,** is the most common form of diabetes and affects 6% of the population. Typical onset occurs after the age of 40, which explains why it has also been known as "adult onset" diabetes. There appears to be a genetic tendency because it runs in families. Obesity is also a common factor.

Symptoms begin gradually and include the three "polys": **polydipsia, polyuria, and polyphagia.** The person often notes the ability to eat more than usual yet lose weight.

Diagnosis may involve several tests, but the GTT is the most common and is considered diagnostic for diabetes. With this test, the patient eats or drinks a specific quantity of carbohydrates; the blood glucose level is checked at specified intervals of time afterward. An abnormally high rise in blood glucose indicates the body's inability to utilize the glucose efficiently. In NIDDM, the pancreas still produces *some* insulin. The problem may be a deficiency of insulin production or resistance to the insulin that is produced.

Case Study Questions

1. Marsha experienced which of the following symptoms prior to diagnosis?
   a. Decreased appetite
   b. Decreased urination
   c. Decreased visual acuity
   d. Weight gain

2. Marsha's diagnosis of type II diabetes was confirmed by:
   a. A test that measured blood glucose levels at specified intervals after ingestion of glucose
   b. Testing a drop of capillary blood obtained by pricking the finger
   c. Testing her blood after a 12-hour fast
   d. A test that reveals the average blood glucose level over the past 3 to 4 months

3. Which of the following statements is true regarding NIDDM?
   a. It is the second most common form of diabetes
   b. Onset is usually before the age of 40 years
   c. Obesity is uncommon
   d. There may be a genetic component

4. Which of the following statements is true regarding NIDDM?
   a. The pancreas fails to produce insulin
   b. The body may be resistant to the insulin that is produced
   c. Exercise is not recommended for disease management
   d. The primary form of treatment is injection of insulin

WEB SITES

American Diabetes Association: www.diabetes.org
Endocrine Society: www.endo-society.org
American Thyroid Association: www.thyroid.org

PREFIX AND SUFFIX REVIEW

Tables 9-4 and 9-5 contain a review of selected prefixes and suffixes. Refer to these tables as necessary when you complete the practice exercises at the end of the chapter.

TABLE 9-4
PREFIX PRONUNCIATIONS AND MEANINGS

Prefix	Pronunciation Guide	Meaning
an-	ăn	without, absence of
dys-	dĭs	painful, difficult
eu-	ū	good, normal
hyper-	hī-pĕr	excessive, above normal
hypo-	hī-pō	below normal, beneath
poly-	pŏl-ē	many, much

TABLE 9-5
SUFFIX PRONUNCIATIONS AND MEANINGS

Suffix	Pronunciation Guide	Meaning
-ic, tic	ĭk, tĭk	pertaining to
-dipsia	dĭp-sē-ă	thirst
-dynia	dĭn-ē-ă	pain
-cele	sēl	hernia
-centesis	sĕn-tē-sĭs	surgical puncture
-edema	ĕ-dē-mă	swelling

(continues on page 210)

SUFFIX PRONUNCIATIONS AND MEANINGS *(Continued)*

Suffix	Pronunciation Guide	Meaning
-emia	ē-mē-ă	a condition of the blood
-ism	ĭzm	condition
-itis	ī-tĭs	inflammation
-logist	lō-jĭst	specialist in the study of
-meter	mĕ -tĕr	instrument for measuring
-oma	ō-mă	tumor
-pathy	pă-thē	disease
-penia	pē-nē-ă	deficiency
-pepsia	pĕp-sē-ă	digestion
-phagia	fā-jē-ă	eating, swallowing
-phasia	fā-zē-ă	speech
-rrhaphy	ră-fē	suture, suturing
-rrhexis	rĕk-sĭs	rupture
-therapy	thēr-ă-pē	treatment
-uria	ū-rē-ă	urine

PRACTICE EXERCISES

Complete the following practice exercises. The answers can be found in Appendix G.

Matching

Match the following combining forms with the correct meanings. Some answers may be used more than once or not at all.

Exercise A

1. _____ thym/o
2. _____ orchi/o
3. _____ calc/o
4. _____ orch/o

     a.   toxin, poison
     b.   thyroid
     c.   water
     d.   ovary

5. _____ hydr/o   e. parathyroid

6. _____ orchid/o   f. gland

7. _____ thyroid/o   g. testes

8. _____ test/o   h. thymus

9. _____ toxic/o   i. calcium

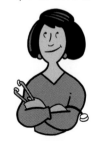

"You're off to a
solid start. Keep
up the effort!"

Exercise B

1. _____ parathyroid/o   a. pancreas

2. _____ ovari/o   b. gland

3. _____ aden/o   c. sugar, glucose

4. _____ pancreat/o   d. adrenal

5. _____ adrenal/o   e. parathyroid

6. _____ oophor/o   f. water

7. _____ adren/o   g. ovary

8. _____ gluc/o   h. thyroid

9. _____ glyc/o

Word Building

*Using **only** the word parts in the lists provided, create medical
terms with the indicated meanings.*

Prefixes	**Combining Forms**	**Suffixes**
an-	aden/o	-centesis
eu-	adrenal/o	-emia
hyper-	calc/o	-ic
hypo-	gluc/o	-ism
	hydr/o	-itis
	oophor/o	-logist
	orch/o	-meter
	pancreat/o	-oma
	parathyroid/o	-pathy

thym/o   -therapy
thyroid/o
toxic/o

1. specialist in the study of poison _____

2. tumor of the gland _____

3. below normal parathyroid (hormone) _____

4. adrenal disease _____

5. excessive calcium in the blood _____

6. instrument used to measure glucose _____

7. water treatment _____

8. surgical puncture of the ovary _____

9. condition of absent testes _____

10. inflammation of the pancreas _____

11. pertaining to a normal thymus _____

12. condition of excessive thyroid _____

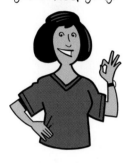

"This is hard, I know, but you're doing great! Keep going!"

Deciphering Terms

Write the correct translation of the following medical terms.

1. pancreatic _____

2. ovariocele _____

3. orchidodynia _____

4. adrenopathy _____

5. orchiorrhaphy _____

6. euglycemia _____

7. dysthymic _____

8. thyroidorrhexis _____

9. adenopathy _____

10. glucopenia _____

11. hypoglycemia _____

True or False

Decide whether the following statements are true or false.

1. True   False   The abbreviation **TSH** stands for thyroid-stimulating hormone.

2. True   False   The abbreviation **ADH** stands for adenopathy.

3. True   False   The abbreviation **K** stands for kidney.

4. True   False   A **glucose tolerance test** measures blood glucose levels at specified intervals after ingestion of glucose.

5. True   False   The abbreviation **Na** stands for natural.

6. True   False   A **glycosylated hemoglobin** test reveals the average blood glucose level over the past 9 months.

7. True   False   The abbreviation **fsbs** stands for fasting blood sugar.

8. True   False   A **TSH** level may be drawn to check for hypothyroidism.

9. True   False   The abbreviation **PTH** stands for parathyroid hormone.

10. True   False   A **fasting blood sugar** is drawn after a 12-hour fast.

11. True   False   **Retinopathy** is a disease of the kidneys.

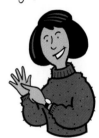

"You're over halfway there. Keep up the great work!"

Fill in the Blank

Fill in the blanks below.

1. The abbreviation *BS* stands for _____ _____.

2. Chester has a condition caused by hyposecretion of growth hormone during his childhood. He has

   _____.

3. The abbreviation *CA* stands for _____.

4. The abbreviation *Ca* stands for _____.

5. The thyroid hormones include _____

   and _____.

6. The abbreviation for diabetes mellitus is

   _____.

7. There are two major forms of diabetes. One is *NIDDM*, which stands for _____ _____ _____ _____.

8. Another form of diabetes is *IDDM*, which stands for _____

   _____ _____ _____.

9. The abbreviation *GH* stands for _____ _____.

10. Abnormal protrusion of the eyeballs is known as

    _____.

11. Lonnie has a condition caused by hypersecretion of growth hormone during his childhood. He has

    _____.

12. Adreanna has exopthalmos caused by hyperthyroidism. She has _____ _____.

13. _____ _____ is a condition caused by hypersecretion of glucocorticoids by the adrenal gland, which results in altered fat distribution and muscle weakness.

14. Benito has developed nonpitting edema in connective tissues caused by advanced hypothyroidism. He has

_____.

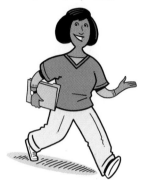

"You're almost to the finish line. Don't stop now."

15. Julia has _____ disease, which results in destruction of the adrenal cortex.

16. _____ is a condition of arrested physical and mental development caused by insufficient thyroid secretion.

Common Diagnostic Tests

Write the definition of the following diagnostic tests.

1. **Fasting blood glucose (FBG):**

2. **Finger stick blood sugar (fsbs):**

3. **Glucose tolerance test (GTT):**

4. **Glycosylated hemoglobin (Hbg A1c):**

5. **Thyroid-stimulating hormone (TSH):**

Multiple Choice Questions

Select the one best answer to the following multiple choice questions.

1. Annette Vizzetti has insulin-dependent diabetes mellitus (IDDM). She is a regular patient at Valley Clinic and has come in today for a regular health check. The physician is interested in knowing what Annette's average blood glucose levels have been for the last 3 to 4 months. Which of the following tests is the physician most likely to order?

   a. TSH

   b. GTT

   c. Hbg A1c

   d. Fasting blood glucose

2. When Annette Vizzetti was first diagnosed with diabetes, she came to see her physician, complaining of the three "polys," the classic signs of diabetes. Which of the following is NOT one of them?

   a. Polyphagia

   b. Polydipsia

   c. Polyphasia

   d. Polyuria

3. Normal blood glucose level is 70 to 120. When Annette Vizzetti checks her glucose today, she notes that the result is 182. The correct medical term for this condition is:

   a. Hypercalcemia

   b. Hyperglycemia

   c. Hyperkalemia

   d. Hypernatremia

4. Ms. Singh has been ill for the past 2 days with stomach flu. Her symptoms include diarrhea and vomiting. She has not been able to keep food or fluids down and has become moderately dehydrated. Because of her diarrhea and poor

intake, her blood potassium level is below normal. The correct term for this is:

a. Hyponatremia

b. Hypocalcemia

c. Hypokalemia

d. Hypoglycemia

5. Because Ms. Singh is dehydrated, her blood sodium level is higher than normal. The correct term for this is:

a. Hypernatremia

b. Hypercalcemia

c. Hyperkalemia

d. Hyperglycemia

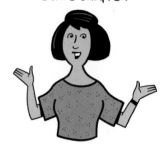

"Congratulations! You've completed the entire chapter!"

MUSCULOSKELETAL SYSTEM

STRUCTURE AND FUNCTION OF THE SKELETAL SYSTEM

The muscular and skeletal systems work together in a complementary fashion to make movement possible. Neither one would be effective without the other. The bones of the skeletal system provide a strong framework for the muscles that are attached to them. When the muscles contract and relax in different combinations, they create a pulling effect on the bones that results in movement.

The skeletal system provides strength and protection for soft tissues and organs (Fig. 10-1). For example, the **cranium** provides a strong protective container for the brain. The **vertebral column** protects the spinal cord and combines with the **sternum** and **ribs** to create the **thorax,** which protects the heart, great vessels, and the lungs (Fig. 10-2).

The skeletal system also plays important roles in blood production and mineral regulation. Blood cells are produced within the bone marrow. This explains why a **bone marrow transplant** may be necessary for someone with a blood disorder such as leukemia. Minerals, such as calcium and magnesium, that are stored in bones are largely responsible for providing their strength and hardness. These same minerals are necessary for nerve and muscle function, so they must be present in these tissues as well as in the blood. If mineral levels are too low, the body takes minerals from the bones, which may result in decreased bone strength and density. If sufficient minerals are not replenished, the result is a disorder known as **osteoporosis.**

Bones are dynamic, living, ever-changing structures. Unlike the white, dry, dead bones you may have seen, living bones have a rich supply of blood vessels and nerves. If injured, they may hurt and

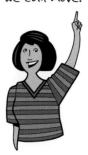

"Muscles and bones work together so that we can move."

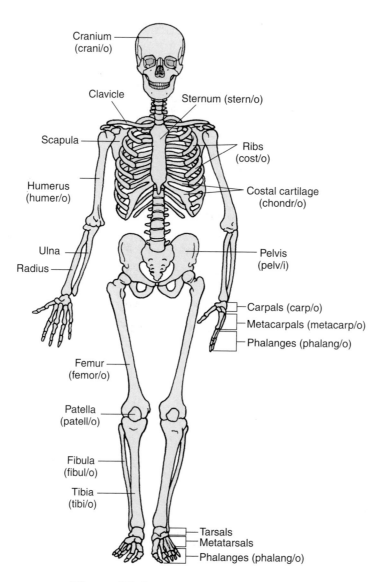

Cranium
(crani/o)

Clavicle

Sternum (stern/o)

Scapula

Ribs
(cost/o)

Humerus
(humer/o)

Costal cartilage
(chondr/o)

Ulna

Radius

Pelvis
(pelv/i)

Carpals (carp/o)

Metacarpals (metacarp/o)

Phalanges (phalang/o)

Femur
(femor/o)

Patella
(patell/o)

Fibula
(fibul/o)

Tibia
(tibi/o)

Tarsals
Metatarsals
Phalanges (phalang/o)

Figure 10-1   The skeletal system.

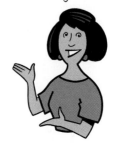

"The skeletal system protects soft tissues and organs."

"Weight-bearing exercise helps bones become stronger."

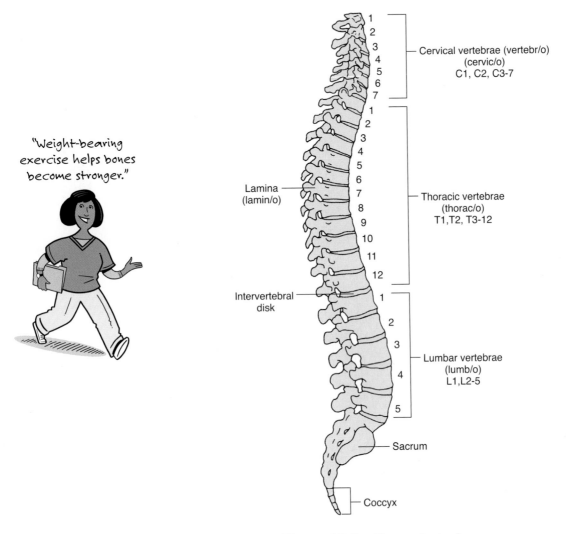

Figure 10-2   The vertebral column.

bleed. This also means they have the ability to heal themselves. The most common injuries to bones are fractures. Important to the healing process is the development of **osteocytes,** new bone cells, which are constantly created through **osteogenesis.** New cells replace older ones that are injured or broken down as they age. Because bones are able to remodel themselves in this way, certain activities such as weight-lifting or weight-bearing exercise like jogging and walking stimulate the bones to become stronger and denser.

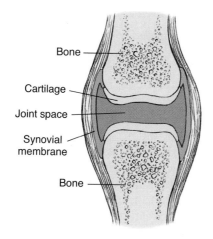

Figure 10-3 Synovial joint.

A *joint* is a place where two bones meet. There are several types of joints in the body. Joints are held together and stabilized by fibrous bands of tissue known as **ligaments.** Some joints allow for a great deal of movement, such as the shoulder joint. Some allow no movement, such as those between the bones of the skull. The movable joints are similar and include structures located within a *joint capsule* (Fig. 10-3). These structures include the **articular cartilage,** the **synovial membrane,** and the **synovial fluid.** They protect bone ends and facilitate movement. A common disorder of these joints is called **osteoarthritis,** also known as **degenerative joint disease (DJD),** which causes erosion of these structures, resulting in inflammation, pain, and decreased movement.

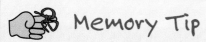 Memory Tip

Memorize all of the vertebrae with these three simple steps. First, memorize the following numbers in the same way you might memorize a phone number: 7, 12, 5, 5, 4. Second, memorize the order of the vertebra from the most superior (top) to the most inferior (bottom): cervical, thoracic, lumbar, sacral, coccyx. Third, pair them up (7-cervical, 12-thoracic, 5-lumbar, 5-sacral and 4-coccyx). You have now memorized 33 of the bones in the body—the vertebrae!

STRUCTURE AND FUNCTION OF THE MUSCULAR SYSTEM

Muscles are attached to bones by strong bands of fibrous connective tissue known as **tendons.** Muscles serve three important functions in the body: movement, support, and heat production.

Muscles generally work together in muscle groups to achieve movement and stabilization. For example, the quadriceps femoris, or "quads" as they are commonly known, work together to extend the leg. While this is occurring, other muscles in the trunk of the body maintain enough muscle contraction to keep the body in a stable, upright position.

"Heat is a natural by-product of muscle activity."

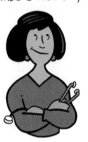

A great deal of energy is expended to keep the muscles working. A natural by-product of this expenditure is heat. This is why a person feels hot and begins to perspire while exercising. The body has produced more heat than is needed, and natural cooling mechanisms kick in. This same principle works when a person is exposed to a cold environment and more body heat is needed. Without adequate clothing, body temperature drops and shivering begins. Shivering is an involuntary action of the muscles that results in heat energy as a by-product, which warms the body.

There are three types of muscles: voluntary or skeletal, involuntary or visceral, and cardiac. Skeletal muscles may be controlled voluntarily by conscious thought. They move body parts, implement reflexive movement, and maintain posture. Involuntary muscles are found in visceral organs, such as the stomach and intestines. They are not under voluntary control. Cardiac muscle is found only in the heart and is discussed in Chapter 4. Figure 10-4 illustrates the major muscles of the body.

COMBINING FORMS

Table 10-1 contains combining forms that pertain to the musculoskeletal system along with examples of terms which utilize the combining form, and a pronunciation guide. Read out loud to yourself as you move from left to right across the table. Be sure to use the pronunciation guide so that you can learn to say the terms correctly.

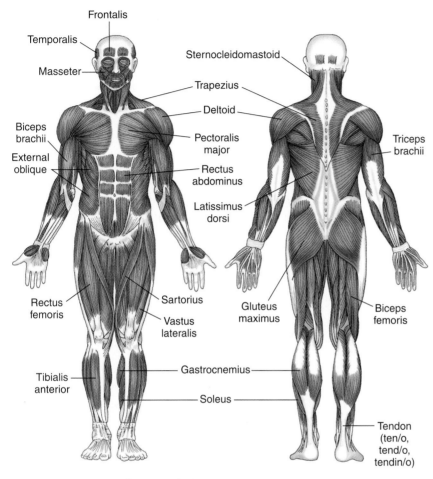

Figure 10-4 The muscular system.

TABLE 10-1

COMBINING FORMS RELATED TO THE MUSCULOSKELETAL SYSTEM

Combining Form	Meaning	Example (Pronunciation)	Meaning of New Term
arthr/o	joint	arthrocentesis (ăr-thrō-sĕn-TĒ-sĭs)	surgical puncture of a joint
carp/o	carpus	carpectomy (kăr-PĔK-tō-mē)	surgical removal of a carpus

(continues on page 224)

223

COMBINING FORMS RELATED TO THE MUSCULOSKELETAL SYSTEM (*Continued*)

Combining Form	Meaning	Example (Pronunciation)	Meaning of New Term
cervic/o	neck	cervicodynia (sĕr-vĭ-kō-DĬN-ē-ă)	pain in the neck
chondr/o	cartilage	chondrodysplasia (kŏn-drō-dĭs-PLĀ-zē-ă)	difficult or painful (abnormal) cartilage development
cost/o	ribs	costochondritis (kŏs-tō-kŏn DRĪ-tĭs)	inflammation of the ribs and cartilage
crani/o	cranium	craniocerebral (krā-nē-ō-sĕr-Ē-brăl)	pertaining to the cranium and brain
femor/o	femur	femorotibial (fĕm-ō-rō-TĬB-ē-ăl)	pertaining to the femur and tibia
fibul/o	fibula	fibular (FĬB-ū-lăr)	pertaining to the fibula
humer/o	humerus	humeral (HŪ-mĕr-ăl)	pertaining to the humerus
lamin/o	lamina	laminectomy (lăm-ĭ-NĔK-tō-mē)	surgical removal of the lamina
lumb/o	lower back	lumbodynia (lŭm-bō-DĬN-ē-ă)	pain in the lower back
metacarp/o	metacarpus	metacarpectomy (mĕt-ă-kăr-PĔK-tō-mē)	surgical removal of the metacarpus
myel/o	spinal cord, bone marrow	myeloplegia (mī-ĕl-ō-PLĒ-jē-ă)	paralysis of the spinal cord
my/o	muscle	myocardial (mī-ō-KĂR-dē-ăl)	pertaining to heart muscle
orth/o	straight	orthopnea (or-THŎP-nē-ă)	breathing straight (upright)
oste/o	bone	osteolytic (ŏs-tē-ō-LĬT-ĭk)	pertaining to destruction of the bone
patell/o	patella	patellapexy (pă-TĔL-ă-pĕk-sē)	surgical fixation of the patella
pelv/i	pelvis	pelvimeter (pĕl-VĬM-ĕ-tĕr)	instrument for measuring the pelvis
phalang/o	phalanges	phalangitis (făl-ăn-JĬ-tĭs)	inflammation of the phalanges

Combining Form	Meaning	Example (Pronunciation)	Meaning of New Term
stern/o	sternum	sternocostal (stĕr-nō-KŎS-tăl)	pertaining to the sternum and ribs
ten/o	tendon	tenodynia (tĕn-ō-DĬN-ē-ă)	pain in a tendon
tend/o		tendotome (TĔN-dō-tōm)	instrument used to cut a tendon
tendin/o		tendinous (TĔN-dĭ-nŭs)	pertaining to a tendon
thorac/o	thorax	thoracolumbar (thō-răk-ō-LŬM-bar)	pertaining to the thorax and lower back
tibi/o	tibia	tibiofibular (tĭb-ē-ō-FĬB-ū-lăr)	pertaining to the tibia and fibula
vertebr/o	vertebrae	vertebroplasty (vĕr-TĒ-brō-plăs-tē)	surgical repair of the vertebrae

STOP HERE.
Remove the Combining Form Flash Cards for Chapter 10, and run through them at least 3 times before you continue.

PRACTICE EXERCISES

Use Table 10-1 to fill in the answers below.

1. _____ pertaining to the tibia and fibula

2. _____ inflammation of the phalanges

3. _____ surgical repair of the vertebrae

4. _____ surgical fixation of the patella

5. _____ pain in a tendon

6. _____ pertaining to the femur and tibia

7. _____ instrument used to cut a tendon

8. _____ pertaining to a tendon

9. _____ paralysis of the spinal cord

10. _____ surgical removal of the lamina

11. _____ surgical removal of the metacarpus

12. _____ pertaining to the humerus

13. _____ pertaining to the sternum and ribs

14. _____ instrument for measuring the pelvis

15. _____ pain in the lower back

16. _____ breathing straight (upright)

17. _____ pertaining to heart muscle

18. _____ surgical puncture of a joint

19. _____ surgical excision of a carpus

20. _____ difficult or painful (abnormal) cartilage formation or growth

21. _____ inflammation of the ribs and cartilage

22. _____ pain in the neck

23. _____ pertaining to the cranium and brain

24. _____ pertaining to the fibula

25. _____ pertaining to destruction of the bone

26. _____ pertaining to the thorax and lower back

27. Fill in the blanks with the appropriate anatomical term and/or combining form.

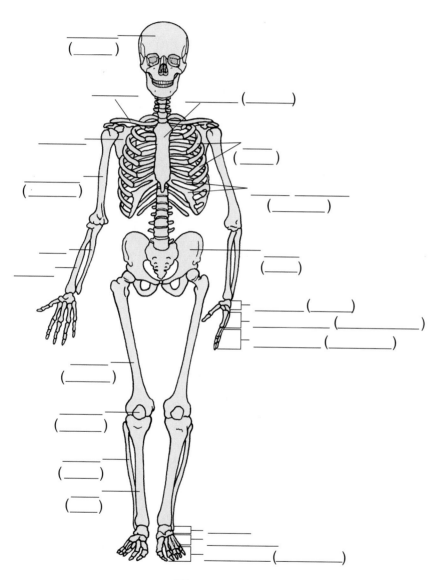

Figure 10-5

28. Fill in the blanks with the appropriate anatomical term and/or combining form.

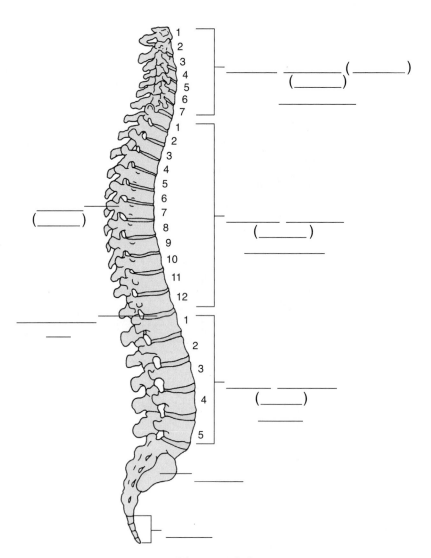

Figure 10-6

29. Fill in the blanks with the appropriate anatomical term and/or combining form.

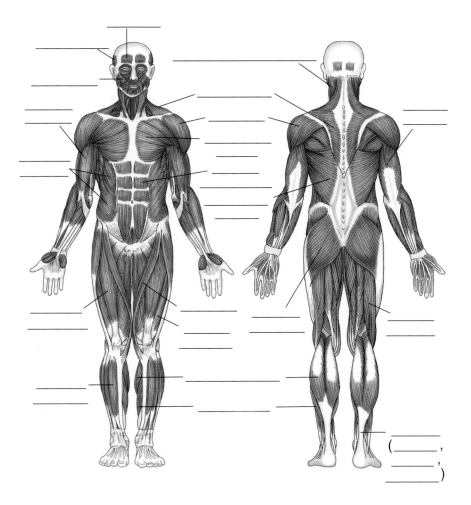

Figure 10-7

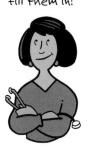

"Looks kind of empty without labels. Let's fill them in!"

ABBREVIATIONS

Table 10-2 lists some of the most common abbreviations related to the musculoskeletal system as well as others often used in medical documentation.

TABLE 10-2	
ABBREVIATIONS	
AKA	above the knee amputation
AP	anterioposterior
BKA	below the knee amputation
C1-C7	1st cervical vertebra, 2nd cervical vertebra, etc.
DJD	dengenerative joint disease (osteoarthritis)
Fx	fracture (Fig. 10-8)
IM	intramuscular
L1-L5	1st lumbar vertebra, 2nd lumbar vertebra, etc.
ortho	orthopedic or straight
RA	rheumatoid arthritis
S1-S5	1st sacral vertebra, 2nd sacral vertebra, etc.
T1-T12	1st thoracic vertebra, 2nd thoracic vertebra, etc.
THR	total hip replacement
TKR	total knee replacement

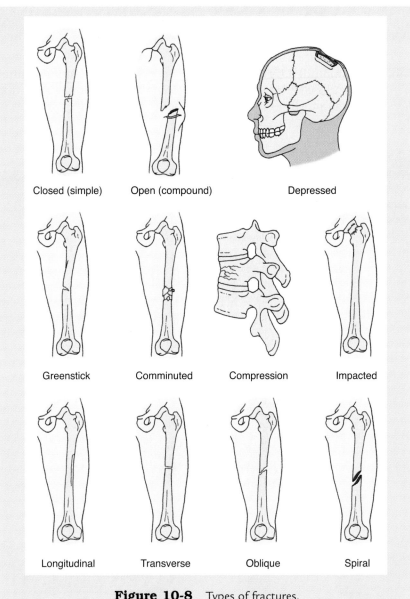

Closed (simple)   Open (compound)   Depressed

Greenstick   Comminuted   Compression   Impacted

Longitudinal   Transverse   Oblique   Spiral

Figure 10-8   Types of fractures.

STOP HERE.

Remove the Abbreviation Flash Cards for Chapter 10, and run through them at least 3 times before you continue.

PATHOLOGY TERMS

Table 10-3 includes terms that relate to diseases or abnormalities of the musculoskeletal system. Use the pronunciation guide, and say the terms out loud as you read them. This will help you get in the habit of saying them properly.

TABLE 10-3	
PATHOLOGY TERMS	
carpal tunnel syndrome (CTS)	compression of median nerve causes pain or numbness in the wrist, hand, and fingers (Fig. 10-9)

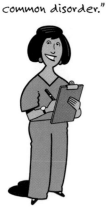

"With so many people using computers, CTS has become a common disorder."

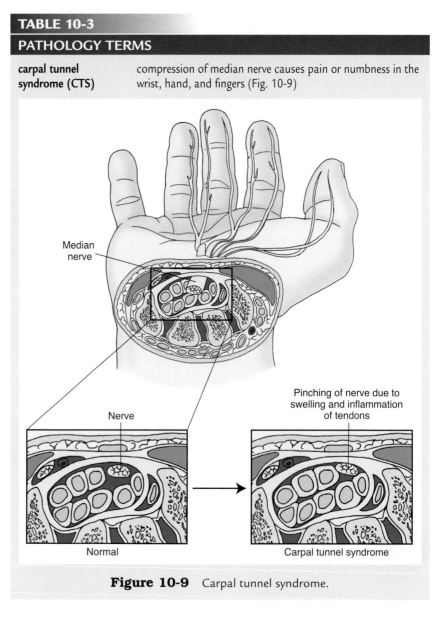

Figure 10-9   Carpal tunnel syndrome.

contracture (kŏn-TRĂK-chūr)	fibrosis of connective tissue which decreases mobility of a joint
crepitation (krĕp-ĭ-TĀ-shŭn)	a grating sound from broken bones or a clicking or crackling sound from joints
gout (gowt)	hereditary form of arthritis characterized by uric acid accumulation in the joints, especially in the great toe
herniated (hĕr-nē-Ā-tĕd) **disk**	herniation of the soft center of an intervertebral disk between two vertebrae (Fig. 10-10)

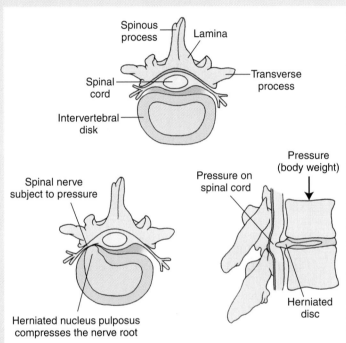

Figure 10-10   Herniated disk.

kyphosis (kī-FŌ-sĭs)	abnormal increase in curvature of thoracic vertebrae, causing "hunchback" (Fig. 10-11)
lordosis (lor-DŌ-sĭs)	abnormal increase in curvature of lumbar vertebrae causing "swayback" (see Fig. 10-11)
muscular dystrophy (DĬS-trō-fē) **(MD)**	hereditary, progressive, terminal disease that causes muscle atrophy and death, usually by age 20
myasthenia gravis (mī-ăs-THĒ-nē-ă GRĂV-ĭs)	autoimmune motor disorder that causes progressive muscle fatigue and weakness
osteoarthritis (ŏs-tē-ō-ăr-THRĪ-tĭs)	type of arthritis marked by progressive cartilage deterioration in synovial joints and vertebrae

(continues on page 234)

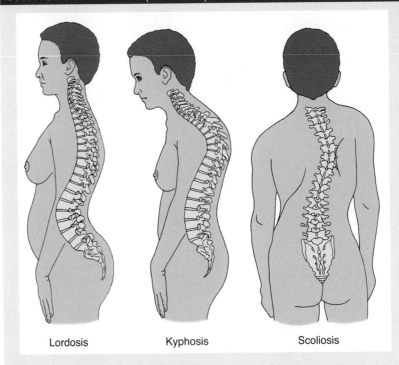

Lordosis   Kyphosis   Scoliosis

Figure 10-11 Abnormal curvature of the spine.

rheumatoid arthritis (RA) (ROO-mă-toyd ăr-THRĪ-tĭs)	autoimmune form of arthritis that causes pain and deformity of joints and may affect organ systems (Fig. 10-12)

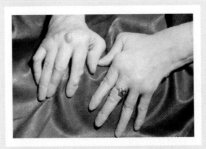

Figure 10-12 Rheumatoid arthritis. (From Dillon PM: Nursing Health Assessment. Philadelphia, FA Davis, p 627.)

scoliosis (sko-lē-Ō-sĭs)	abnormal S-shaped, lateral curvature of the vertebrae (see Fig. 10-11)
sprain (sprān)	complete or incomplete tear in ligaments around a joint
strain (strān)	injury to muscle or tendon

STOP HERE.
Remove the Pathology Term Flash Cards for Chapter 10, and run through them at least 3 times before you continue.

COMMON DIAGNOSTIC TESTS

Bone marrow aspiration: bone marrow specimen is removed from the cortex of a flat bone for analysis

Bone scan: a gamma camera is used to detect abnormalities in bone density after injection of radioactive material

Creatine kinase (CK): isoenzyme in skeletal and cardiac muscle released into the blood when muscle cells are damaged

Electromyogram (EMG): records electrical activity of skeletal muscles; used to diagnose neuromuscular disorders

Erythrocyte sedimentation rate (ESR) or "sed" rate: rate at which red blood cells settle in a tube of unclotted blood; an elevated ESR indicates inflammation

Rheumatoid factor: a blood test used to identify rheumatoid arthritis

CASE STUDY

Read the following case study, and answer the questions that follow. Most of the terms are included in this chapter. Refer to the Glossary or to your medical dictionary for the other terms.

Osteoarthritis
Michael Mayhew is a 59-year-old man with osteoarthritis of the knees. He has a history of bilateral knee injuries from college football as well as a 33-year career in construction. He has noticed a slow onset of symptoms, primarily over the past 10 years. His primary complaints were arthralgia and stiffness, especially first thing in the morning. Initial treatment was conservative and included rest, nonsteroidal anti-inflammatory drugs (NSAIDs), physical therapy, and weight loss of 25 lb. In spite of these measures, Mr. Mayhew continued to experience worsening symptoms over the next few years. Eventually, he underwent bilateral TKRs.

Follow-up note: Eight weeks after surgery, Mr. Mayhew stated he was pain-free and had better use of his knees than he had in years.

(continues on page 236)

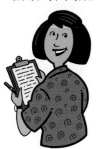

"It's tough to get old, isn't it? Of course, I wouldn't know!"

Osteoarthritis, also known as **degenerative joint disease (DJD),** is the most common form of noninflammatory joint disease. The key feature of DJD is wearing down and loss of cartilage in synovial joints. DJD occurs most often after the age of 40 and involves joints that have had prior injuries or heavy chronic wear and tear. The most common joints involved are those of the hips, knees, hands, and spine. Pathological features include erosion of the articular cartilage, sclerosis of the bone beneath the cartilage, and bone spur formation. The primary symptom is joint pain on weight-bearing. Management of DJD includes rest, NSAIDs, glucosamine supplements, physical therapy, and weight loss (obesity is a common factor). If necessary, the patient may rely on a cane, crutches, or walker. Surgery may eventually be necessary.

Case Study Questions

1. Which of the following statements is true regarding Mr. Mayhew's experience?
    a. He had arthritis in his right knee only
    b. Onset of his arthritis was sudden and severe
    c. His symptoms were worse in the evening
    d. He experienced stiffness in his knees in the mornings

2. What type of surgery did Mr. Mayhew have?
    a. Repair of both knee joints
    b. Replacement of both knee joints
    c. Fixation of both knee joints
    d. Fusion of both knee joints

3. Mr. Mayhew's primary symptom was arthralgia. This means:
    a. Pain in a joint
    b. Inflammation of a joint
    c. Destruction of a joint
    d. Softening of a joint

4. Which of the following statements is true regarding osteoarthritis?
    a. It is an uncommon form of arthritis
    b. It is characterized by demineralization of the bones
    c. It affects joints that have had prior injuries or heavy chronic wear and tear
    d. It most commonly involves the shoulders, elbows, and wrists

WEB SITES

Muscular Dystrophy Association—USA: www.mdausa.org
National Osteoporosis Foundation: www.nof.org
BMC Musculoskeletal Disorders: www.biomedcentral.com/
    bmcmusculoskeletdisord/
Arthritis Foundation: www.arthritis.org/default.asp

PREFIX AND SUFFIX REVIEW

Tables 10-4 and 10-5 contain a review of selected prefixes and suffixes. Refer to these tables as necessary when you complete the practice exercises at the end of the chapter.

TABLE 10-4
PREFIX PRONUNCIATIONS AND MEANINGS

Prefix	Pronunciation Guide	Meaning
extra-	ĕks-tră	away from, external
supra-	soo-pră	excessive, above normal
sub-	sŭb	below normal, beneath
inter	ĭn-tĕr	between
para-	păr-ă	near, surrounding, two like parts

TABLE 10-5
SUFFIX PRONUNCIATIONS AND MEANINGS

Suffix	Pronunciation Guide	Meaning
-al, -ar, -ic, -tic -eal	ăl, ăr, ĭk, tĭk, ē-ăl	pertaining to
-algia -dynia	ăl-jē-ă dĭn-ē-ă	pain
-centesis	sĕn-tē-sĭs	surgical puncture

(continues on page 238)

SUFFIX PRONUNCIATIONS AND MEANINGS *(Continued)*

Suffix	Pronunciation Guide	Meaning
-clasis	klă-sĭs	breaking
-ectomy	ĕk-tō-mē	excision, surgical removal
-itis	ī-tĭs	inflammation
-lysis	lĭ-sĭs	destruction of
-malacia	mă-la-shē-ă	softening
-metry	mĕ-trē	measurement
-oma	ō-mă	tumor
-osis	ō-sĭs	abnormal condition
-pathy	pă-thē	disease
-plasty	plăs-tē	surgical repair
-plegia	plē-jē-ă	paralysis
-pnea	nē-ă	breathing
-ptosis	tō-sĭs	drooping, prolapse
-tome	tōm	cutting instrument
-tomy	tō-mē	cutting into, incision

"Checking your answers AFTER you've completed these exercises provides immediate feedback that will reinforce your learning."

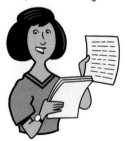

PRACTICE EXERCISES

Complete the following practice exercises. The answers can be found in Appendix G.

Matching

Match the following combining forms with the correct meanings. Some answers may be used more than once or not at all.

Exercise A

1. _____ arthr/o

2. _____ oste/o

3. _____ cost/o

a. spinal cord, bone marrow

b. straight/upright

c. lower back

4. _____ tibi/o   d. lamina

5. _____ lamin/o   e. humerus

6. _____ orth/o   f. rib

7. _____ lumb/o   g. joint

8. _____ cervic/o   h. neck

9. _____ carp/o   i. tibia

10. _____ my/o   j. carpus

11. _____ myel/o   k. muscle

12. _____ humer/o   m. bone

Exercise B

1. _____ patell/o   a. metacarpus

2. _____ thorac/o   b. cartilage

3. _____ pelv/i   c. femur

4. _____ vertebr/o   d. thorax

5. _____ tendin/o   e. cranium

6. _____ chondr/o   f. pelvis

7. _____ tend/o   g. tibia

8. _____ femor/o   h. vertebrae

9. _____ crani/o   i. sternum

10. _____ ten/o   j. patella

11. _____ stern/o   k. phalanges

12. _____ phalang/o   l. tendon

13. _____ metacarp/o

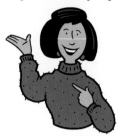

"You're making great progress! Keep going!"

Word Building

*Using **only** the word parts in the lists provided, create medical terms with the indicated meanings.*

Prefixes	Combining Forms	Suffixes
inter-	arthr/o	-al
para-	carp/o	-ar
sub-	cervic/o	-algia
	chondr/o	-dynia
	cost/o	-ectomy
	crani/o	-itis
	femor/o	-malacia
	humer/o	-metry
	lamin/o	-oma
	lumb/o	-pathy
	metacarp/o	-plasty
	myel/o	-plegia
	my/o	-pnea
	orth/o	-tome
	oste/o	
	patell/o	
	pelv/i	
	phalang/o	
	stern/o	
	tendin/o	
	thorac/o	
	tibi/o	
	vertebr/o	

1. pertaining to the ribs and vertebrae _____

2. inflammation of the bone and joint _____

3. pertaining to the carpus _____

4. pertaining to near or beside the neck _____

5. cartilage pain _____

6. instrument used to cut the lamina _____

7. pertaining to between the ribs _____

8. surgical repair of the skull _____

9. pertaining to the femur _____

10. pertaining to the humerus _____

11. breathing straight (upright) _____

12. pain in the lower back _____

13. inflammation of the metacarpus _____

14. tumor of the bone marrow or spinal
    cord _____

15. paralysis of the muscle _____

16. pertaining to beneath the sternum _____

17. disease of the bones _____

18. surgical removal of the patella _____

19. measurement of the pelvis _____

20. inflammation of the phalanges _____

21. inflammation of the tendon _____

22. pertaining to the thorax and lower
    back _____

23. softening of the tibia _____

24. surgical repair of the vertebrae _____

Deciphering Terms

Write the correct translation of the following medical terms.

1. paravertebral _____

2. supratibial _____

3. thoracic _____

4. tendolysis _____

5. sternotomy _____

6. phalangeal _____

7. patelloptosis _____

8. osteotomy _____

9. myopathy _____

10. myelosclerosis _____

11. lumbar _____

12. laminotomy _____

13. femorodynia _____

14. craniotomy _____

15. costochondritis _____

16. cervicitis _____

17. carpocentesis _____

18. arthralgia _____

19. osteoclasis _____

20. extratibial _____

"You're halfway there. Keep up the great work!"

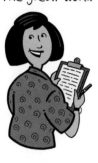

True or False

Decide whether the following statements are true or false.

1. True   False   **BKA** is an abbreviation for broken.

2. True   False   **Gout** is a hereditary from of arthritis characterized by uric acid accumulation in the joints, especially in the great toe.

3. True   False   The abbreviation **IM** stands for immobility.

4. True   False   A **contracture** is fibrosis of connective tissue, which decreases mobility of a joint.

5. True   False   **Muscular dystrophy** is a hereditary, progressive, terminal disease that causes muscle atrophy and death.

6. True   False   **Lordosis** is an abnormal increase in curvature of lumbar vertebrae, causing "swayback."

7. True   False   The abbreviation **RA** stands for rheumatoid arthritis.

8. True   False   A **sprain** is an injury to muscle or tendon.

9. True   False   **Kyphosis** is an abnormal increase in curvature of thoracic vertebrae, causing "hunchback."

10. True   False   **Myasthenia gravis** is a grating sound from broken bones or a clicking or crackling sound from joints.

Fill in the Blank

Fill in the blanks below.

1. When the lower leg is removed below the knee, the procedure is known as a(n) _____ _____ _____ _____, abbreviated as _____.

2. Suzanne has an abnormal S-shaped, lateral curvature of her spine. This condition is known as _____.

3. Another name for degenerative joint disease is _____.

4. A(n) _____ is an injury to muscle or tendon.

5. Joseph has _____, which causes progressive cartilage deterioration in synovial joints and vertebrae.

6. The cervical vertebrae are abbreviated

_____.

7. When Howard climbs the stairs, his knees creak. This crackling sound is known as _____.

8. Lorinda spends much of her workday at a computer; as a result, she has developed _____ _____ _____, which is due to compression of the median nerve and causes pain and numbness in her wrist, hands, and fingers.

9. The abbreviation for Lorinda's disorder

is _____.

10. Two common types of major joint replacement are

_____ _____ _____ and

_____ _____ _____.

11. The sacral vertebrae are abbreviated

_____.

12. The combining form *orth/o* stands for

_____ or _____.

13. Pablo had a(n) _____ of his radius and ulna and had to have his forearm in a cast for several weeks. The abbreviation for this is _____.

14. The physician ordered a(n) _____ x-ray, which will aim from front to back. This is abbreviated

_____.

15. The lumbar vertebrae are abbreviated

    _____.

16. Sylvester had severe back pain after an accident at work.
    The physician has diagnosed him with a(n) _____
    _____, which is the herniation of the soft center of an
    intervertebral disk between two vertebrae.

17. The thoracic vertebrae are abbreviated

    _____.

18. An autoimmune form of arthritis that causes pain and
    deformity of joints and may involve organ systems is
    _____ arthritis.

19. When the leg is removed from above the knee, it is known as
    a(n) _____ _____ _____ _____
    and is abbreviated as _____.

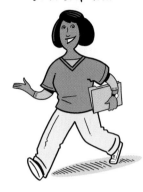

"You're almost done.
Don't stop now!"

COMMON DIAGNOSTIC TESTS

Write the definition of the following diagnostic tests.

1. **Bone marrow aspiration:**

2. **Bone scan:**

3. **Creatine kinase (CK):**

4. **Electromyogram (EMG):**

5. **Erythrocyte sedimentation rate (ESR) or "sed" rate:**

6. **Rheumatoid factor:**

Multiple Choice Questions

Select the one best answer to the following multiple choice questions.

1. Which of the following conditions is responsible for compression of the median nerve, resulting in pain or numbness in wrist, hand, and fingers?

   a. Herniated disk

   b. Myasthenia gravis

   c. Gout

   d. Carpal tunnel syndrome

2. Which of the following conditions is an autoimmune motor disorder that causes progressive muscle fatigue and weakness?

   a. Myasthenia gravis

   b. Gout

   c. Carpal tunnel syndrome

   d. Kyphosis

3. Martha Snyder has been diagnosed with rheumatoid arthritis. She most likely has which of the following complaints?

   a. Arthralgia

   b. Osteoplegia

   c. Patelloptosis

   d. Metacarpotome

4. Jose Fernandez has carpal tunnel syndrome. He most likely has which of the following symptoms?

   a. Phalangodynia

   b. Carpotomy

   c. Fibulitis

   d. Patellitis

5. Ilka Heidrick has myasthenia gravis. Which of the following is she most likely to experience?

   a. Increased energy level after exercise

   b. Progressive dementia

   c. Arthralgia

   d. Progressive fatigue

"You've completed the entire chapter. What a great accomplishment!"

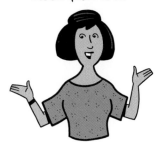

11

SPECIAL SENSES (EYES AND EARS)

STRUCTURE AND FUNCTION OF THE EYES

The eyes are the sensory organs of sight. The **pupil** functions as an adjustable window that lets light into the inner structures of the eye (Fig. 11-1). Just behind the pupil is the **lens**, which focuses the light and sends it to the **retina** at the back of the eyeball. The retina translates the information into nerve impulses that are sent to the brain by way of the **optic nerve.** The brain interprets these data as visual images and then determines their meaning and significance.

In order to see clear, sharp images, the lens must change shape constantly with the help of the tiny **ciliary muscles.** With age, the lens loses its elasticity and is less able to accommodate for distance changes, especially close-up viewing. Because of this, many people need glasses when they reach their 40s. The corrective lens is able to make up for what the eye's natural lens can no longer do.

The eyeballs are located within the orbital cavity and are surrounded by protective structures. These include the eyebrows, eyelashes, and eyelids, which help keep foreign objects out of the eye. If an object gets past this defense system, it is quickly washed away by the fluid commonly known as tears, which contain a bacteria-killing enzyme.

"The eye's natural lens loses elasticity with age, causing loss of visual acuity."

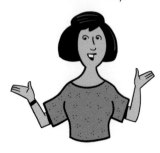

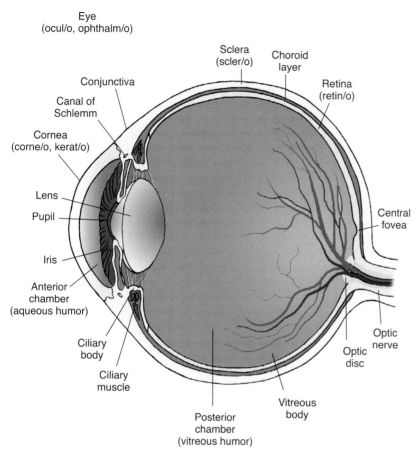

Eye
(ocul/o, ophthalm/o)

Sclera
(scler/o)

Choroid
layer

Retina
(retin/o)

Conjunctiva

Canal of
Schlemm

Cornea
(corne/o, kerat/o)

Lens

Pupil

Iris

Anterior
chamber
(aqueous humor)

Ciliary
body

Ciliary
muscle

Posterior
chamber
(vitreous humor)

Vitreous
body

Optic
disc

Optic
nerve

Central
fovea

Figure 11-1   The eye.

STRUCTURE AND FUNCTION OF THE EARS

The ears are responsible for hearing and have the ability to collect and transmit sound waves to the brain for interpretation. Ears also play an important role in maintaining balance and equilibrium. The structures of the ears are located in three main areas: the external, middle, and internal ear (Fig. 11-2).

"Swimmer's ear, also known as otitis externa, is an infection of the external ear canal."

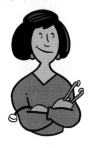

Ear (ot/o)

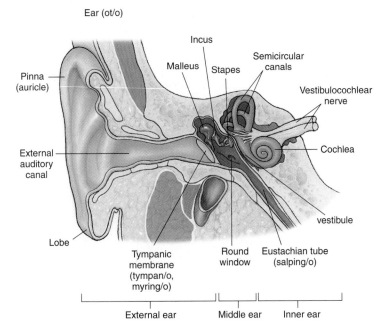

Figure 11-2 The ear.

"When your ears 'pop,' air is moving through the eustachian tube to equalize pressure."

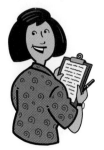

The **external ear** is composed of the **auricle,** which is the outer structure; the **ear canal,** also called the auditory canal; and the **tympanic membrane (TM),** commonly known as the eardrum. Infections of the external ear are called **otitis externa**, also known as swimmer's ear, and are common in children in the summer when they spend a great deal of time in the water. When the ear canal harbors moisture, it creates a warm, hospitable environment conducive to fungal and bacterial growth.

The **middle ear** begins just inside the tympanic membrane and includes the three tiny bones called the **malleus, incus,** and **stapes.** They transmit sound vibrations from the tympanic membrane to the structures within the inner ear. The **eustachian tube** connects the middle ear to the throat and allows air movement back and forth to equalize air pressure. When the eustachian tube is closed and middle ear pressure is greater or less than atmospheric pressure, a person may describe the ear as feeling "plugged." The pressure is relieved when the eustachian tube opens to allow air through. This is a common experience with altitude changes and explains the "ear popping" sensation when you travel over the mountains or ride in an airplane.

The **inner ear** includes the **semicircular canals, vestibule,** and **cochlea.** These structures receive sound waves and translate them into nerve impulses that are sent to the brain via the **auditory nerve (vestibulocochlear).** The anatomy of the inner ear is quite complex, with a mazelike design of twists and turns. Because of this, the inner ear is sometimes also called the **labyrinth.** Inflammation of the inner ear is much less common than that of the middle or outer ear. It is called **labyrinthitis** and causes a very unpleasant sensation known as **vertigo.** This happens because the inner ear also contains special structures for the maintenance of balance and equilibrium.

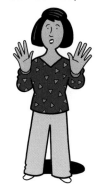

"Vertigo is an unpleasant sensation of spinning or movement in space."

COMBINING FORMS

Table 11-1 contains combining forms that pertain to the special senses, examples of terms that utilize the combining forms, and a pronunciation guide. Read out loud to yourself as you move from left to right across the table. Be sure to use the pronunciation guide so you can learn to say the terms correctly.

TABLE 11-1
COMBINING FORMS RELATED TO SPECIAL SENSES

Combining Form	Meaning	Example (Pronunciation)	Meaning of New Term
acous/o	hearing	acoustic (ă-KOOS-tĭk)	pertaining to hearing
audi/o		audiometry (aw-dē-ŎM-ĕ-trē)	measurement of hearing
blephar/o	eyelid	blepharoptosis (blĕf-ă-rō-TŌ-sĭs)	drooping or prolapse of the eyelid
corne/o	cornea	corneous (KOR-nē-ŭs)	pertaining to the cornea
kerat/o		keratocele (kĕr-ĂT-ō-sēl)	herniation of the cornea
dipl/o	double	diploid (DĬP-loyd)	resembling double
myring/o	tympanic membrane	myringoplasty (mĭr-ĬN-gō-plăst-ē)	surgical repair of the tympanic membrane
tympan/o		tympanosclerosis (tĭm-pă-nō-sklĕ-RŌ-sĭs)	hardening of the tympanic membrane
ocul/o	eye	oculomycosis (ŏk-ū-lō-mī-KŌ-sĭs)	abnormal condition of eye fungus
ophthalm/o		ophthalmorrhexis (ŏf-thăl-mō-RĔK-sĭs)	rupture of the eye

(continues on page 252)

COMBINING FORMS RELATED TO SPECIAL SENSES *(Continued)*

Combining Form	Meaning	Example (Pronunciation)	Meaning of New Term
ot/o	ear	otorrhea (ō-tō-RĒ-ă)	flow or discharge from the ear
retin/o	retina	retinopexy (rĕt-ĭn-ō-PĔK-sē)	surgical fixation of the retina
salping/o	tube (eustachian, fallopian)	salpingopharyngeal (săl-pĭng-gō-fă-RĬN-jē-ăl)	pertaining to the eustachian tube and pharynx
scler/o	sclera, hardening	scleral (sklĕ-ăl)	pertaining to the sclera

STOP HERE.

Remove the Combining Form Flash Cards for Chapter 11, and run through them at least 3 times before you continue.

PRACTICE EXERCISES

Use Table 11-1 to fill in the answers below.

1. _____ flow or discharge from the ear

2. _____ rupture of the eye

3. _____ abnormal condition of eye fungus

4. _____ hardening of the tympanic membrane

5. _____ pertaining to hearing

6. _____ measurement of hearing

7. _____ herniation of the cornea

8. _____ surgical fixation of the retina

9. _____ pertaining to the sclera

10. _____ drooping or prolapse of the eyelid

11. _____ pertaining to the eustachian tube
and pharynx

12. _____ pertaining to the cornea

13. _____ resembling double

14. _____ surgical repair of the tympanic
membrane

15. Fill in the blanks with the appropriate anatomical term
and/or combining form.

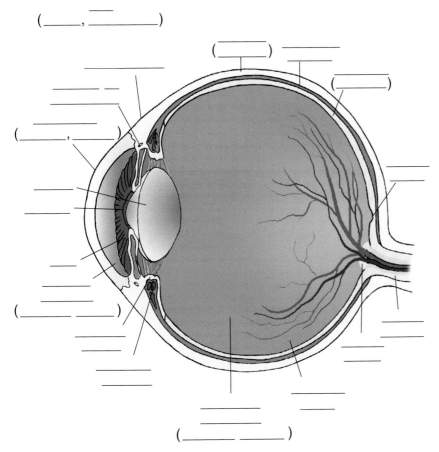

Figure 11-3

16. Fill in the blanks with the appropriate anatomical term and/orcombining form.

___ (___)

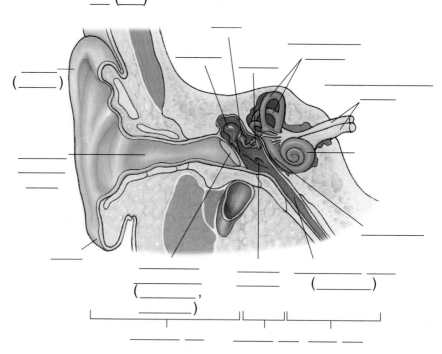

Figure 11-4

ABBREVIATIONS

Table 11-2 lists some of the most common abbreviations related to the special senses.

TABLE 1-2	
ABBREVIATIONS	
Eye	
EOM	extraocular movement
PERRLA	pupils are equal, round, reactive to light and accommodation
Ear	
EENT	eyes, ears, nose, and throat
ENT	ears, nose, and throat

STOP HERE.
Remove the Abbreviation Flash Cards for Chapter 11, and run through them at least 3 times before you continue.

PATHOLOGY TERMS

Table 11-3 includes terms that relate to diseases or abnormalities of the special senses. Use the pronunciation guide, and say the terms out loud as you read them. This will help you get in the habit of saying them properly.

"Diabetic retinopathy is a leading cause of blindness."

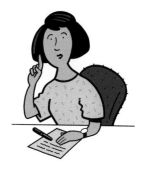

TABLE 11-3
PATHOLOGY TERMS

Eye

astigmatism (ă-STĬG-mă-tĭzm)	abnormal curvature of the cornea that distorts the visual image
cataract (KĂT-ă-răkt)	cloudiness of the lens due to protein deposits
conjunctivitis (kŏn-jŭnk-tĭ-VĪ-tĭs)	inflammation of the conjunctiva, also called pink eye
diabetic retinopathy (dī-ă-BĔT-ĭk rĕt-ĭn-ŎP-ă-thē)	loss of vision due to microvascular changes caused by diabetes
glaucoma (glaw-KŌ-mă)	vision loss caused by increased intraocular pressure
hordeolum (hor-DĒ-ō-lŭm)	infection of a sebaceous gland of the eyelid, also called a sty (Fig. 11-5)
macular (MĂK-ū-lăr) **degeneration**	breakdown of the macula, resulting in loss of central vision
retinal (RĔT-ĭ-năl) **detachment**	separation of the retina, resulting in blindness (if not corrected)
strabismus (stră-BĬZ-mŭs)	deviated direction of the eyes (Fig. 11-6)

(continues on page 256)

Eye

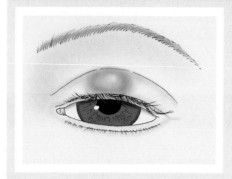

Figure 11-5 Hordeolum (stye).

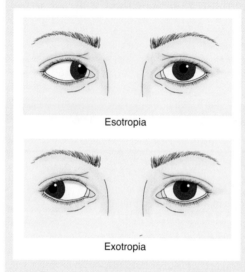

Esotropia

Exotropia

Figure 11-6 Strabismus.

Ear

acute otitis media (AOM) (ō-TĪ-tĭs MĒ-dē-ă)	middle ear infection
anacusis (ăn-ă-KŪ-sĭs)	total deafness
Meniere's (mān-ē-ĀRZ) **disease**	labyrinth disorder that leads to progressive hearing loss, vertigo, and tinnitus
otosclerosis (ō-tō-sklē-RŌ-sĭs)	ossification of structures of the inner ear, causing progressive hearing loss
presbycusis (prĕz-bĭ-KŪ-sĭs)	age-related hearing loss
tinnitus (tĭn-Ī-tŭs)	ringing in the ears
vertigo (VĔR-tĭ-gō)	a feeling of spinning or movement in space

STOP HERE.
Remove the Pathology Term Flash Cards for Chapter 11, and
run through them at least 3 times before you continue.

COMMON DIAGNOSTIC TESTS

Tonometry: measurement of intraocular pressure

Snellen's eye chart: vision screening tool that contains rows of
letters in decreasing size

Weber's test: a screening test for hearing that evaluates bone
conduction using a tuning fork (Fig. 11-7)

Rinne's test: a screening test for hearing that compares bone
conduction to air conduction using a tuning fork (Fig. 11-8)

Audiometric tests: detailed hearing tests conducted by an
audiologist

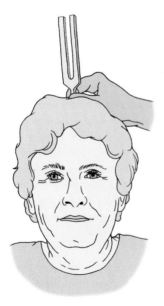

Figure 11-7   Weber's test.

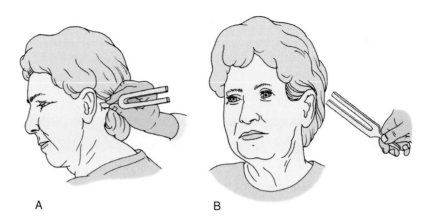

A   B

Figure 11-8   Rinne's test.

CASE STUDY

Read the following case study, and answer the questions that follow. Most of the terms are included in this chapter. Refer to the Glossary or to your medical dictionary for the other terms.

Acute Otitis Media (AOM)

Brad Stephens is a 5-year-old child with a Hx of chronic otitis media. With his first ear infection at 9 months of age, his symptoms were quite pronounced. He spiked a 104.5°F fever, ate and slept poorly, and was extremely fussy. However, with repeated episodes of AOM as he has aged, his symptoms have lessened significantly, making it difficult for his parents to know when he has an ear infection. Often his only symptom is fussiness. Brad has responded reasonably well in the past to antibiotics and decongestants, yet the infections frequently recur a short time later. Now at the age of 5, he still has one to two episodes of AOM each month. This raises concerns about hearing loss, and so he was referred to an ENT specialist for consultation. The result has been the decision to perform bilateral tympanotomy with tube placement.

Acute otitis media, the most common infection in infants and children, occurs when bacteria make their way from the oropharynx into the middle ear via the eustachian tube. Infections such as AOM often occur near the end of an upper respiratory infection (URI). Tissues are inflamed and edematous, and secretions are copious. Other risk factors for OM include allergies and sinusitis. As infection sets in, the middle ear becomes inflamed, which causes edema and pressure in the middle ear. Serous fluid usually accumulates behind the tympanic membrane (TM) as well. In some children, the eustachian tube does not readily open to allow passage of air or fluid to relieve this pressure. As a result, the TM begins to bulge outward. This pressure along with the inflammation causes pain and a sensation of the ear being "plugged." Hearing is temporarily impaired at this point. In severe cases, the TM becomes blistered or even ruptures, which results in scarring and varying amounts of hearing loss.

With mild cases of OM, treatment may focus on relieving pain with analgesics such as acetaminophen and treating congestion. More severe cases are treated with antibiotics. In the case of chronic OM, surgery is considered. Surgery is generally a last resort and serves the purpose of "buying time" while the child grows and matures. In many cases, a child will outgrow ear infections as the structures of the middle ear and throat further develop and the eustachian tube begins to work more effectively.

When a tympanotomy is performed, tiny tubes are inserted into the TM, which creates a windowlike opening between the middle and outer ear. This does not prevent OM from occurring. However, it does allow fluid and air to escape, reducing pressure in the middle ear and preventing rupture of the TM. This reduces the risk of permanent damage or hearing loss. An added advantage is that it becomes easier to recognize an infection because drainage from the ear is easily observed. This allows for earlier treatment. The tiny tubes remain in place for 6 months to 2 years, eventually working their way out into the ear canal, at which time the TM heals itself.

"Small children can experience ear pain on an airplane due to the effects of changing air pressure on the developing eustachian tubes."

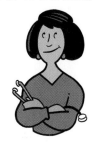

Case Study Questions

1. Which of the following statements is true regarding Brad's experience?
   a. His symptoms worsened over time
   b. Brad was referred to a physician who specialized in disorders of the ears, nose, and throat
   c. Brad did not respond well to antibiotic therapy
   d. His parents could easily tell when Brad had an ear infection

2. Brad underwent a bilateral tympanotomy with tube placement. This procedure involves:
   a. Excision and removal of the eardrums
   b. Replacing the eardrums with tubes
   c. Creation of a mouthlike opening into the eustachian tube
   d. Cutting into the eardrums to place tubes

(continues on page 260)

3. Which of the following statements is true regarding AOM?
   a. It is an uncommon type of infection in infants and children
   b. It is contagious
   c. It is caused when a virus attacks the middle ear
   d. It is caused by bacterial growth in the middle ear

4. Which of the following factors contribute to the development of AOM?
   a. A dry environment
   b. Failure of the outer ear canal to develop and work properly
   c. Allergies and sinusitis
   d. Accumulation of fluid in front of the TM

5. Which of the following statements is true regarding treatment of AOM?
   a. Antibiotics are always prescribed
   b. Decongestants may be used
   c. Surgery is common
   d. Analgesics are seldom used

6. Which of the following statements is true regarding the surgical procedure that Brad underwent?
   a. The purpose was to buy some time while the structures in his ear and throat further developed
   b. The purpose was to repair the defect in his middle ear and cure his problem
   c. The purpose was to restore his lost hearing
   d. The purpose was to prevent the occurrence of OM

7. Which of the following statements is true regarding the tubes that are placed in the TM?
   a. They will be surgically removed once the ear has healed
   b. They allow for the escape of fluid or air
   c. They force the eustachian tube to work properly
   d. They usually remain in place for 5 years

WEB SITES

American Foundation for the Blind (AFB): www.afb.org
American Academy of Ophthalmology: www.aao.org
Glaucoma Research Foundation: www.glaucoma.org
The Ear Foundation: www.earfoundation.org
American Society for Deaf Children: www.deafchildren.org

PREFIX AND SUFFIX REVIEW

Tables 11-4 and 11-5 contain a review of selected prefixes and suffixes. Refer to these tables as necessary when you complete the practice exercises at the end of the chapter.

TABLE 11-4
PREFIX PRONUNCIATIONS AND MEANINGS

Prefix	Pronunciation Guide	Meaning
a-, an-	ă, ăn	without, absence of
hyper-	hī-pĕr	excessive, above normal
intra-	ĭn-tră	within, inner
neo-	nē-ō	new
retro-	rĕt-rō	behind, back

TABLE 11-5
SUFFIX PRONUNCIATIONS AND MEANINGS

Suffix	Pronunciation Guide	Meaning
-al, -ar, -ic, -ous	ăl, ăr, ĭk, ŭs	pertaining to
-edema	ĕ-dē-mă	swelling
-itis	ĭ-tĭs	inflammation
-kinesia	kĭ-nē-zē-ă	movement
-logy	lō-jē	study of
-metry	mĕ-trē	measurement
-oid	oyd	resembling
-opia	ō-pē-ă	vision
-osis	ō-sĭs	abnormal condition
-pathy	pă-thē	disease
-phobia	fō-bē-ă	fear
-plasia	plā-zē-ă	formation, growth
-plasty	plăs-tē	surgical repair
-plegia	plē-jē-ă	paralysis
-ptosis	tō-sĭs	drooping, prolapse
-scope	skōp	instrument to view
-tomy	tō-mē	cutting into, incision

PRACTICE EXERCISES

Complete the following practice exercises. The answers can be found in Appendix G.

Matching

Match the following prefixes with the correct meanings. Some answers may be used more than once or not at all.

Exercise A

1. _____ tympan/o

2. _____ kerat/o

3. _____ ocul/o

4. _____ ophthalm/o

5. _____ blephar/o

6. _____ myring/o

7. _____ corne/o

a. eye

b. cornea

c. hardening, sclera

d. eyelid

e. tympanic membrane

f. retina

g. tube

h. ear

i. hearing

"You're off to a great start. Keep up the great effort!"

Exercise B

1. _____ salping/o

2. _____ retin/o

3. _____ dipl/o

4. _____ ot/o

5. _____ acous/o

6. _____ scler/o

7. _____ audi/o

a. hearing

b. eye

c. hardening, sclera

d. tube

e. eyelid

f. double

g. retina

h. ear

Word Building

*Using **only** the word parts in the lists provided, create medical terms with the indicated meanings.*

Prefixes	**Combining Forms**	**Suffixes**
an-	acous/o	-edema
hyper-	audi/o	-itis
intra-	blephar/o	-logy
neo-	corne/o	-opia
	dipl/o	-osis
	myring/o	-ous
	ocul/o	-pathy
	ophthalm/o	-plasia
	ot/o	-plasty
	retin/o	-scope
	salping/o	-ic
	scler/o	-tomy

1. pertaining to absence of hearing _____

2. new growth _____

3. swelling of the eyelid _____

4. far vision _____

5. study of hearing _____

6. inflammation of the cornea _____

7. double vision _____

8. cutting into the tympanic membrane _____

9. instrument for viewing the eye _____

10. disease of the retina _____

11. surgical repair of the sclera _____

12. surgical repair of the eyes _____

13. pertaining to the ears _____

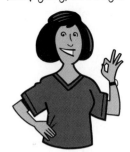

"You're doing awesome! Keep going, mi amigo!"

Deciphering Terms

Write the correct translation of the following medical terms.

1. keratoid _____

2. neoplasia _____

3. myringomycosis _____

4. tympanometry _____

5. retro-ocular _____

6. ophthalmoplegia _____

7. otoplasty _____

8. oculonasal _____

9. tympanic _____

10. keratotomy _____

11. blepharoptosis _____

12. ophthalmokinesia _____

13. intraocular _____

True or False

Decide whether the following statements are true or false.

1. True   False   The abbreviation **ENT** stands for eyes, ears, nose, and throat.

2. True   False   **Conjunctivitis** is a condition of inflammation of the conjunctiva.

3. True   False   The abbreviation **EOM** stands for extraocular movement.

4. True   False   **Tinnitus** is a feeling of dizziness or vertigo.

5. True   False   **Strabismus** is a condition of blindness.

6. True   False   **Otosclerosis** causes progressive hearing loss.

7. True   False   **Vertigo** is ringing in the ears.

8. True   False   **Acute otitis media** is an infection of the outer ear.

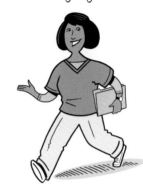

"You learn by repetition, so keep going!"

Fill in the Blank

Fill in the blanks below.

1. Dr. Strouse specializes in treating *EENT* disorders. Therefore, she treats disorders of the _____, _____, _____, and

   _____.

2. When Dr. Strouse charts *PERRLA*, it means _____

   _____ _____, _____, _____

   _____ _____ and _____.

3. Kari wears corrective lenses because she has an abnormal curvature of the cornea that distorts her visual image. This is known as a(n) _____.

4. Herbert has total deafness. The term for this is

   _____.

5. Hilda has hearing loss due to her advanced age. The term for this is _____.

6. Jack has _____ _____, which is a disorder of the inner ear that causes progressive hearing loss, vertigo, and tinnitus.

7. _____ causes vision loss due to increased intraocular pressure.

8. David is a farmer who has developed cloudiness of the lens due to protein deposits. This is called _____.

9. Monty has been a diabetic for 20 years and is developing the signs of _____ _____, which is vision loss due to his diabetes.

10. Blake is losing his central vision due to a breakdown of the macula. This is known as _____ _____.

11. Louise has an inflammation of one of the sebaceous glands of her eyelid. This is known as _____.

12. Dennis has a separation of the retina that has caused blindness in his left eye. This is known as _____ _____.

Common Diagnostic Tests

Write the definition of the following diagnostic tests.

1. **Tonometry:**

2. **Snellen's eye chart:**

3. **Weber's test:**

4. **Rinne's test:**

5. **Audiometric tests:**

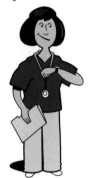

"You've nearly completed the chapter. Keep up the great work!"

Multiple Choice Questions

Select the one best answer to the following multiple choice questions.

1. Which of the following conditions does NOT result in vision loss?

   a. Presbycusis

   b. Diabetic retinopathy

   c. Retinal detachment

   d. Glaucoma

2. Which of the following conditions results in abnormal curvature of the cornea that distorts the visual image?

   a. Presbycusis

   b. Astigmatism

   c. Cataract

   d. Hordeolum

3. Albert Mills is an elderly man who has totally lost his hearing due to advanced age. This condition is known as:

   a. Photophobia

   b. Glaucoma

   c. Presbycusis

   d. Hordeolum

4. A type of blindness caused by diabetes is known as diabetic
   _____.

   a. Retinopathy

   b. Cataract

   c. Macular degeneration

   d. Meniere's disease

5. Onset of blindness caused by increased intraocular pressure is known as:

   a. Cataract

   b. Macular degeneration

   c. Hordeolum

   d. Glaucoma

"Congratulations! You've completed the last chapter! What a fantastic accomplishment!"

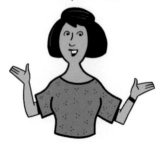

ABBREVIATIONS

SYMBOLS

♂	male
♀	female

A

Abd	abdomen
ABGs	arterial blood gases
ADH	antidiuretic hormone
AIDS	acquired immunodeficiency syndrome
AKA	above the knee amputation
ALS	amyotrophic lateral sclerosis (Lou Gehrig disease)
AP	anteroposterior
APTT (PTT)	activated partial thromboplastin time
ARDS	acute respiratory distress syndrome
ASHD	atherosclerotic heart disease

B

bid	twice a day
BKA	below the knee amputation
BP	blood pressure
BPH	benign prostatic hypertrophy
BRP	bathroom privileges
BM	bowel movement
BS	blood sugar
Bx	biopsy

C

$\bar{c}$	with
C1-C7	1st cervical vertebra, 2nd cervical vertebra, etc.
Ca, CA	calcium, cancer
CABG	coronary artery bypass graft
CAD	coronary artery disease
CHF	congestive heart failure
CNS	central nervous system
CO_2	carbon dioxide
c/o	complaint/complains of
COPD	chronic obstructive pulmonary disease
CPR	cardiopulmonary resuscitation
C-section	cesarean section
C&S	culture and sensitivity
CSF	cerebrospinal fluid
CT	computed tomography
CV	cardiovascular
CVA	cerebrovascular accident

D

D&C	dilation and curettage
DJD	degenerative joint disease (osteoarthritis)

DM	diabetes mellitus
Dx	diagnosis

E

EENT	eyes, ears, nose, and throat
EEG	electroencephalography
EGD	esophagogastroduodenoscopy
EKG	electrocardiogram
EMG	electromyogram
ENT	ears, nose, and throat
EOM	extraocular movement
ERCP	endoscopic retrograde cholangiopancreatography
ESRD	end-stage renal disease

F

FBS	fasting blood sugar
FH	family history
fsbs	finger stick blood sugar
Fx	fracture

G

GERD	gastroesophageal reflux disease
GH	growth hormone
GI	gastrointestinal
GTT	glucose tolerance test
GU	genitourinary
Gyn	gynecology

H

h, hr	hour
HIV	human immunodeficiency virus
HTN	hypertension
Hx	history

I

IBD	inflammatory bowel disease
IBS	irritable bowel syndrome

I&D	incision and drainage
ID	intradermal (injection)
IDDM	insulin dependent diabetes mellitus (type I diabetes)
IM	intramuscular
INR	international normalized ratio
IUD	intrauterine device
IV	intravenous
IVF	in vitro fertilization
IVP	intravenous pyelogram

K

K	potassium
KUB	kidney, ureter, bladder

L

L1-L5	1st lumbar vertebra, 2nd lumbar vertebra, etc.
LA	left atrium
LFTs	liver function tests
LMP	last menstrual period
LP	lumbar puncture
LV	left ventricle

M

MI	myocardial infarction
MRI	magnetic resonance imaging
MS	multiple sclerosis

N

Na	sodium
NG	nasogastric
NIDDM	noninsulin-dependent diabetes mellitus (type II diabetes)
N&V	nausea and vomiting
NPO	nothing by mouth

O

O_2	oxygen
OB-GYN	obstetrics and gynecology
OC	oral contraceptives
ortho	orthopedic
OTC	over the counter

P

PAP	Papanicolaou smear
PCP	*Pneumocystis carinii* pneumonia
PE	physical examination
PERRLA	pupils are equal, round, reactive to light and accomodation
PID	pelvic inflammatory disease
PND	paroxysmal nocturnal dyspnea
PNS	peripheral nervous system
PO	by mouth
PR	per rectum
PTCA	percutaneous transcoronary angioplasty
PTH	parathyroid hormone
PTT	partial thromboplastin time
PUD	peptic ulcer disease

Q

qam	every morning
qh	every hour
qhs	every evening (hour of sleep)
qid	four times a day
q2h	every 2 hours

R

RA	rheumatoid arthritis, right atrium
ROM	range of motion
RP	retrograde pyelogram
RV	right ventricle

S

S1-S5	1st sacral vertebra, 2nd sacral vertebra, etc.
$\bar{s}$	without
SARS	sudden acute respiratory syndrome
SBO	small bowel obstruction
SOB	short of breath
stat	immediately
STD	sexually transmitted disease
Sx	symptoms

T

T1-T12	1st thoracic vertebra, 2nd thoracic vertebra, etc.
T3, T4	thyroid hormones
TAH-BSO	total abdominal hysterectomy, bilateral salpingo-oophorectomy
TB	tuberculosis
THR	total hip replacement
tid	three times a day
TKR	total knee replacement
TSH	thyroid stimulating hormone
TURP	transurethral resection of the prostate
Tx	treatment

U

UA	urinalysis
UGI	upper gastrointestinal
URI	upper respiratory infection
UTI	urinary tract infection

V

VC	vital capacity
VD	venereal disease

DISCONTINUED ABBREVIATIONS

The following abbreviations may be found in current medical records. However, the use of these terms is strongly discouraged because of the high rate of errors in transcription or interpretation.

Inappropriate Abbreviation	Rationale	Replace With
AD: right ear	mistaken for AS, AU, OS, OD, OU	write "right ear"
AS: left ear	mistaken for AD, AU, OS, OD, OU	write "left ear"
AU: both ears	mistaken for AS, AD, OS, OD, OU	write "both ears"
cc: cubic centimeter	mistaken for U (units) when poorly written	write "ml" for milliliters
dc, DC, D/C: discharge or discontinue	mistaken for each other	write either "discharge" or "discontinue" depending on which is most accurate (e.g., discharge a patient, discontinue a medication)
MS, MSO_4: morphine, morphine sulfate	mistaken for magnesium sulfate	write "morphine sulfate"
$MgSO_4$: magnesium sulfate	mistaken for morphine sulfate	write "magnesium sulfate"
OD: right eye	mistaken for AS, AU, AD, OS, OU	write "right eye"
OS: left eye	mistaken for AS, AU, AD, OD, OU	write "left eye"
OU: both eyes	mistaken for AS, AU, AD, OS, OD	write "both eyes"
qd: every day	mistaken for every other day	write "daily"
qod: every other day	mistaken for every day or 4 times per day	write "every other day"
SC or SQ: subcutaneous	mistaken for SL (sublingual) or "5 every"	write: "Sub-Q," "SubQ," or "subcutaneously"
µg: microgram	mistaken for milligram (results in 1000 times overdose!)	write "mcg"
u: unit	when written poorly is mistaken as zero, four, or cc	write "unit"
trailing zero (4.0 mg)	decimal point may be missed, resulting in an overdose of 10 times prescribed amount	never write an unnecessary zero after a decimal point
lack of leading zero (.4 mg)	decimal point may be missed, resulting in a overdose of 10 times prescribed amount	always use a zero before a decimal point to indicate its' presence (0.4 mg)

GLOSSARY OF PATHOLOGY TERMS

A

abrasion (ă-BRĀ-zhŭn): scraping away of skin or mucous membranes

acquired immunodeficiency syndrome (AIDS): caused by human immuno-deficiency virus (HIV), resulting in weakening of immune system

acute respiratory distress syndrome (ARDS): hypoxemia and respiratory failure due to severe inflammatory damage to lungs; occurs after severe infection or trauma

Addison's disease: disorder in which adrenal cortex is destroyed

alopecia (ăl-ō-PĒ-shē-ă): absence or loss of hair

Alzheimer's (ĂLTS-hī-mĕrz) **disease:** a form of chronic, progressive dementia caused by atrophy of brain tissue

anacusis (ăn-ă-KŪ-sĭs): total deafness

aneurysm (ĂN-ū-rĭzm): weakening of the wall of a vessel

arrhythmia (ă-RĬTH-mē-ă): loss of a regular heart rhythm (irregular beat)

ascites (ă-SĪ-tēz): accumulation of serous fluid in the peritoneal (abdominal) cavity

asthma (ĂZ-mă): episodic narrowing and inflammation of the airways in response to various triggers; key symptoms include wheezing, shortness of breath, and cough

astigmatism (ă-STĬG-mă-tĭzm): abnormal curvature of the cornea that distorts the visual image

B

Bell's palsy (PAWL-zē): a form of facial paralysis affecting one or both sides of the face, which is usually temporary

benign prostatic hypertrophy (bē-NĪN prŏs-TĂT-ĭc hī-PĔR-trŏ-fē): enlargement of the prostate gland, common in elderly men

bowel obstruction: A partial or complete blockage of the lumen of the small or large intestine

bruit (brwē): soft blowing sound caused by turbulent blood flow

C

candidiasis (kăn-dĭ-DĪ-ă-sĭs): vaginal fungal infection caused by *Candida albicans;* key symptoms include itching, burning, thick curdy discharge

carpal tunnel syndrome: compression of median nerve causes pain or numbness in wrist, hand, and fingers

cataract (KĂT-ă-răkt): cloudiness of the lens due to protein deposits

cellulitis (sĕl-ū-LĪ-tĭs): bacterial infection of the skin

cerebrovascular (sĕr-ĕ-brō-VĂS-kū-lăr) **accident (CVA):** damage or death of brain tissue caused by interruption of blood supply due to a clot or vessel rupture; also called stroke, apoplexy, or brain attack

273

chlamydia (klă-MĬD-ē-ă): most common sexually transmitted disease; a bacterial vaginal infection caused by *Chlamydia trachomatis*

chronic obstructive pulmonary disease (COPD): Disease in which alveolar air sacs are destroyed and chronic severe shortness of breath results; major cause is smoking

cirrhosis (sĭ-RŌ-sĭs): chronic liver disease characterized by scarring and loss of normal structure

comedo (KŎM-ē-dō): blackhead

congestive heart failure (CHF): heart condition that results in lung congestion and dyspnea

conjunctivitis (kŏn-jŭnk-tĭ-VĪ-tĭs): inflammation of the conjunctiva

contracture (kŏn-TRĂK-chūr): fibrosis of connective tissue that decreases mobility of a joint

contusion (kŏn-TOO-zhŭn): bruise

coryza (kŏ-RĪ-ză): the common cold

crackles: abnormal lung sound heard with a stethoscope; sounds like Rice Krispies

crepitation (krĕp-ĭ-TĀ-shŭn): a grating sound from broken bones or a clicking or crackling sound from joints

cretinism (KRĒ-tĭn-ĭzm): arrested physical and mental development caused by insufficient thyroid secretion

Crohn's disease (krōnz dĭ-ZĒZ): inflammatory bowel disease marked by patches of full-thickness inflammation anywhere in the gastrointestinal tract

croup (croop): acute viral disease, usually in a small child, marked by a barking cough ("seal-like") and respiratory distress

cryptorchidism (krĭpt-ŎR-kĭd-ĭsm): failure or one or both testes to descend into scrotum

Cushing's (KOOSH-ĭngs) **syndrome:** excessive production of glucocorticoids caused by hypersecretion of adrenal gland

cyst (sĭst): fluid or solid-containing pouch in or under the skin

cystic fibrosis (SĬS-tĭk fĭ-BRŌ-sĭs): Fatal genetic disease that causes frequent respiratory infections, increased airway secretions, and chronic obstructive pulmonary disease in children

D

deep vein thrombosis (DVT): development of a blood clot in a deep vein, usually in the legs

diabetic retinopathy (dī-ă-BĔT-ĭk rĕt-ĭn-ŎP-ă-thē): loss of vision caused by diabetes

diabetes (dī-ă-BĒ-tēz) **mellitus:** chronic metabolic disorder in which the pancreas secretes insufficient amounts of insulin or insulin resistance

diuresis (dī-ū-RĒ-sĭs): abnormal secretion of large amounts of urine

diverticulitis (dī-vĕr-tĭk-ū-LĪ-tĭs): when one or more diverticula become inflamed

diverticulosis (dī-vĕr-tĭk-ū-LŌ-sĭs): condition in which small pouches (diverticula) in the intestinal wall, usually the sigmoid colon, form secondary to increased pressure

dwarfism: hyposecretion of growth hormone during childhood resulting in an abnormally small adult

E

ecchymosis (ĕk-ĭ-MŌ-sĭs): discoloration of the skin; a bruise

ectopic (ĕk-TŎ-pĭk) **pregnancy:** fertilized ovum is implanted outside of the uterus, often in the fallopian tube (tubal pregnancy)

eczema (ĔK-zĕ-mă): inflammatory skin disease with redness, itching, and blisters

embolus (ĔM-bō-lŭs): undissolved matter that floats in the blood or lymph current until it occludes a small vessel causing an infarct

emesis (ĔM-ĕ-sĭs): vomiting

empyema (ĕm-pī-Ē-mă): Collection of infected fluid (pus) in the pleural cavity

end-stage renal disease (ESRD): final phase of kidney disease

endometriosis (ĕn-dō-mē-trē-Ō-sĭs): endometrial tissue grows in abnormal sites in lower abdominopelvic area; causes severe dysmenorrhea

enuresis: (ĕn-ū-RĒ-sĭs): involuntary urination, usually during sleep (bedwetting)

epilepsy (ĔP-ĭ-lĕp-sē): brain disorder characterized by recurrent seizures

epistaxis (ĕp-ĭ-STĂK-sĭs): nosebleed

exophthalmos (ĕks-ŏf-THĂL-mōs): abnormal protrusion of the eyeballs

F

fibrillation (fī-brĭl-Ā-shŭn): abnormal quivering of heart muscle fibers instead of an effective heart beat

fibroids (FĪ-broyds): benign uterine tumors

fissure (FĬSH-ūr): small cracklike break in the skin

G

genital warts: sexually transmitted disease, caused by human papillomavirus; causes painless cauliflowerlike warts; a cause of cervical cancer in women

gigantism: hypersecretion of growth hormone during childhood, resulting in an abnormally large adult

gonorrhea (gŏn-ō-RĒ-ă): sexually transmitted disease, caused by *Neisseria gonorrhoeae;* causes inflammation of mucous membranes

gout (gowt): hereditary form of arthritis characterized by uric acid accumulation in the joints, especially those of the great toe

glaucoma (glaw-KŌ-mă): vision loss caused by increased intraocular pressure

glucosuria (gloo-kō-SŪ-rē-ă): sugar in the urine

glycosuria (glĭ-kō-SŪ-rē-ă): sugar in the urine

Grave's disease: hyperthyroidism caused by an autoimmune response; may cause exopthalmos

H

hemothorax (hē-mō-THŌ-răks): blood or bloody fluid collected in pleural cavity

herpes genitalis (HĔRP-ēs jĕn-ĭ-TĂL-ĭs): sexually transmitted disease caused by herpes simplex virus type 2

hernia (HĔR-nē-ă): protrusion of a structure through the wall that normally contains it

herniated (hĕr-nē-Ā-tĕd) disk: herniation of the soft center of an intervertebral disk between two vertebrae

Hodgkin's disease: type of lymphatic cancer

hordeolum (hor-DĒ-ō-lŭm): sty

Huntington's chorea (kō-RĒ-ă): hereditary nervous disorder that leads to bizarre, involuntary movements and dementia

hypertension (hī-pĕr-TĔN-shŭn): blood pressure that is consistently higher than normal, eventually causing damage to vessels and heart

hypoxia (hī-PŎKS-ē-ă): O_2 deficiency

I

impetigo (ĭm-pĕ-TĪ-gō): skin infection marked by yellow to red crusted or pustular lesions

impotence (ĬM-pŏ-tĕns): inability of a male to achieve or maintain erection

incision (ĭn-SĬZH-ŭn): surgical cut in the flesh (made by a scalpel)

interstitial cystitis (ĭn-tĕr-STĬSH-ăl sĭs-TĪ-tĭs): chronic condition of inflammation of the bladder lining

interstitial nephritis (ĭn-tĕr-STĬSH-ăl nĕf-RĪ-tĭs): pathological changes in renal tissue that destroy nephrons and impair kidney function

intussusception (ĭn-tŭ-sŭ-SĔP-shŭn): slipping or telescoping of a portion of the bowel into itself

irritable bowel syndrome: chronic condition characterized by alternating episodes of constipation and diarrhea

ischemia (ĭs-KĒ-mē-ă): temporary reduction in blood supply to a localized area of tissue

J

jaundice (JAWN-dĭs): condition marked by yellow staining of body tissues and fluids as a result of excessive levels of bilirubin in the blood

K

kyphosis (kī-FŌ-sĭs): abnormal increase in curvature of thoracic vertebrae, causing hunchback

L

laceration (lăs-ĕ-RĀ-shŭn): cut or tear in the flesh

lordosis (lor-DŌ-sĭs): abnormal increase in curvature of lumbar vertebrae, causing swayback

lymphosarcoma (lĭm-fō-săr-KŌ-mă): cancer of lymphatic tissue; not related to Hodgkin's disease

M

macule (MĂK-ūl): flat, discolored spot on the skin (such as a freckle)

macular (MĂK-ū-lăr) **degeneration:** breakdown of the macula, resulting in loss of central vision

Meniere's (măn-ē-ĀRZ) **disease:** disorder of the labyrinth of the inner ear that may lead to progressive hearing loss, vertigo, and tinnitus

mononucleosis (mŏn-ō-nū-klē-Ō-sĭs): acute infection due to Epstein-Barr virus; causes sore throat, fever, fatigue, and enlarged lymph nodes

multiple sclerosis (sklĕ-RŌ-sĭs) **(MS):** progressive degenerative disease of the central nervous system that results in the breakdown of the protective myelin cover on nerve cells; causes muscle weakness and loss of coordination

murmur (MŬR-mŭr): abnormal blowing or swishing sound in the heart due to turbulent blood flow or backflow through a leaky valve

muscular dystrophy (DĬS-trō-fē) **(MD):** hereditary, progressive, terminal disease that causes muscle atrophy and death usually by age 20

myasthenia gravis (mī-ăs-THĒ-nē-ă GRĂV-ĭs): autoimmune motor disorder that causes progressive muscle fatigue and weakness

myocardial (mī-ō-KĂR-dē-ăl) **infarction:** death of heart muscle cells due to occlusion of a vessel

myxedema: advanced hypothyroidism; causes dry, waxy edema in various parts of the body

O

otitis media (ŏs-TĪ-tĭs MĒ-dē-ă): middle ear infection

otosclerosis (ō-tō-sklĕ-RŌ-sĭs): progressive deafness due to ossification of structures of the inner ear

P

palsy (PAWL-zē): partial or complete loss of motor function resulting in paralysis

papule (PĂP-ūl): small, raised spot or bump on skin (such as a wart)

Parkinson's disease: progressive, degenerative disorder affecting the part of the brain controlling movement; results in tremors, gait changes and, in some cases, dementia

peptic ulcer (PĔP-tĭk ŬL-sĕr): inflamed lesion in the gastric or duodenal lining

petechia (pē-TĔ-kē-ă): tiny hemorrhagic spot

phimosis (fĭ-MŌ-sĭs): stenosis or narrowing of the foreskin opening

photophobia (fō-tō-FŌ-bē-ă): excessive sensitivity to light

pleural effusion (PLOO-răl ĕ-FŪ-zhŭn): collection of fluid in the pleural cavity

pneumothorax (nū-mō-THŌ-răks): collection of air in the pleural cavity

poliomyelitis (pōl-ē-ō-mĭ-ĕl-Ī-tĭs): inflammation of the spinal cord by a virus, which may result in spinal and muscle deformity and paralysis

presbycusis (prĕz-bĭ-KŪ-sĭs): loss of hearing due to aging

puncture (PŬNK-chūr): hole or wound made by a sharp pointed instrument

pustule (PŬS-tūl): small pus-filled blister

pyelonephritis (pī-ĕ-lō-nĕ-FRĪ-tĭs): inflammation and infection caused by bacterial growth in the renal pelvis

R

renal failure: failure of the kidneys to eliminate fluids and/or wastes from the body effectively

retinal (RĔT-ĭ-năl) **detachment:** separation of the retina, resulting in blindness if not corrected

rheumatoid arthritis (ROO-mă-toyd ăr-THRĪ-tĭs) **(RA):** autoimmune form of arthritis that causes pain and deformity of joints and that may affect organ systems

rhonchi (RŎNG-ī): coarse, gurgley sound heard in the lungs with a stethoscope; usually caused by secretions in the air passages

S

scabies (SKĀ-bēz): contagious skin disease transmitted by the itch mite

scales (skāls): area of skin that is excessively dry and flaky

sciatica (sī-ĂT-ĭ-kă): severe pain that radiates along the path of the sciatic nerve from the buttocks to the foot

shingles (SHĬNG-lz): occurrence of painful herpetic vesicles, usually on the trunk of the body along a peripheral nerve; caused by herpes zoster virus

spina bifida (SPĪ-nă BĪ-fĭd-ă): incomplete closure of the spinal canal, which may result in protrusion of the spinal cord and meninges at birth and that may cause paralysis

sprain (sprān): complete or incomplete tear in ligaments around a joint

sterility (stĕr-ĬL-ĭ-tē): inability to produce offspring

strabismus (stră-BĬZ-mŭs): deviated direction of the eyes

strain (strān): injury to muscle or tendon

stress incontinence: involuntary urination upon physical stress, such as a cough or sneeze

stridor (STRĪ-dor): high-pitched upper airway sound usually heard without a stethoscope; indicates airway obstruction; a medical emergency

stroke (strōk): death of brain cells due to loss of blood supply (cerebrovascular accident [CVA]), also called brain attack

syphilis (SĬF-ĭ-lĭs): sexually transmitted disease; key symptoms include skin lesions; eventually fatal unless treated

T

tinea (TĬN-ē-ă): fungal skin disease occurring on various parts of the body (ringworm)

tinnitus (tĭn-Ī-tŭs): ringing in the ears

transient ischemic (ĭs-KĒ-mĭk) **attack (TIA):** temporary strokelike symptoms caused by brief interruption of blood supply to part of the brain

trichomoniasis (trĭk-ō-mō-NĪ-ă-sĭs): sexually transmitted disease; infestation with parasite *Trichomonas;* key symptoms are vaginitis, urethritis, and cystitis

U

ulcerative colitis (ŬL-sĕr-ā-tĭv kō-LĪ-tĭs): chronic inflammatory disease of the lining of the colon, marked by up to 20 liquid bloody stools per day

uremia (ū-RĒ-mē-ă): increased level of urea or other protein waste products in the blood

urinary retention: retention of urine in the bladder due to inability to urinate

urinary tract infection (UTI): inflammation and infection caused by bacterial growth in the urinary tract, usually the bladder

uterine prolapse (PRŌ-lăps): protrusion of uterus through vaginal opening

V

varicose veins (VĂR-ĭ-kōs vāns): bulging, distended veins due to incompetent venous valves, usually in the legs

vertigo (VĔR-tĭ-gō): sensation of movement or spinning

vesicle (VĔS-ĭ-kl): clear fluid-filled lesion (such as a blister)

vitiligo (vĭt-ĭl-Ī-gō): patchy loss of skin pigmentation

volvulus (VŎL-vū-lŭs): twisting of the bowel on itself, causing obstruction

W

wheeze (hwēz): continuous, somewhat musical sound heard in the lungs, usually with a stethoscope; caused by partial airway obstruction, as with asthma

GLOSSARY OF MEDICAL TERMS

PART I: MEDICAL TO ENGLISH

Prefixes (listed alphabetically)

a-	without, absence of	extra-	away from, external
ab-	away from	hemi-	half
ad-	toward	hyper-	excessive, above normal
an-	without, absence of	hypo-	below normal, beneath
anti-	against	in-	without, absence of
auto-	self	infra-	positioned beneath
bi-	two	inter-	between
brady-	slow	intra-	within, inner
circum-	around	iso-	same, equal
dia-	through, across	mal-	bad, inadequate
dys-	painful, difficult	macro-	large
ec-	out, outside	micro-	small
ecto-	out, outside	multi-	many, much
en-	within, inner	poly-	much, many
endo-	within, inner	neo-	new
epi-	above, upon	oligo-	deficient
eu-	good, normal	para-	near, beside
ex-	away from, external	peri-	near, beside

(continues on page 280)

post-	after, following		supra-	excessive, above normal
pre-	before		tachy-	rapid
pro-	before, forward		tox-	poisonous
quadri-	four		trans-	through or across
re-	behind, back		tri-	three
retro-	behind, back		ultra-	beyond
sub-	below normal, beneath		uni-	one

Suffixes (listed alphabetically)

-ac	pertaining to		-ectomy	excision, surgical removal
-al	pertaining to		-edema	swelling
-algia	pain		-emia	a condition of the blood
-ar	pertaining to		-emesis	vomiting
-ary	pertaining to		-esthesia	sensation
-cele	hernia		-gen	creating, producing
-centesis	surgical puncture		-genesis	creating, producing
-cide	destroying, killing		-gram	record
-cidal	destroying, killing		-graph	recording instrument
-clasis	breaking		-graphy	process of recording
-clast	breaking		-gravida	pregnant woman
-cyte	cell		-ia	condition
-derma	skin		-ic (-tic)	pertaining to
-dipsia	thirst		-ical	pertaining to
-dynia	pain		-iasis	pathological condition or state
-eal	pertaining to		-ism	condition
-ectasis	dilation, expansion		-ist	specialist

-itis	inflammation	-phasia	speech
-kinesia	movement	-phobia	fear
-kinesis	movement	-phoria	feeling
-lith	stone	-plasia	formation, growth
-logist	specialist in the study of	-plasm	formation, growth
-logy	study of	-plasty	surgical repair
-lysis	destruction of	-plegia	paralysis
-malacia	softening	-pnea	breathing
-megaly	enlargement	-ptosis	drooping, prolapse
-meter	instrument for measuring	-rrhage	bursting forth
-metry	measurement	-rrhagia	bursting forth
-oid	resembling	-rrhaphy	suture, suturing
-ole	small	-rrhea	flow, discharge
-oma	tumor	-rrhexis	rupture
-opia	vision	-scope	instrument to view
-ory	pertaining to	-scopy	visual examination
-osis	abnormal condition	-stasis	stopping
-ous (-tous)	pertaining to	-stenosis	narrowing, stricture
-oxia	oxygen	-stomy	mouth-like opening
-paresis	slight or partial paralysis	-therapy	treatment
-pathy	disease	-tome	cutting instrument
-pause	cessation	-tomy	cutting into, incision
-penia	deficiency	-tripsy	crushing
-pepsia	digestion	-trophy	nourishment or growth
-pexy	surgical fixation	-ule	small
-phage	eating, swallowing	-uria	urine
-phagia	eating, swallowing		

Combining Forms (listed alphabetically)

acous/o	hearing	chondr/o	cartilage
aden/o	gland	col/o	colon
adip/o	fat	colon/o	colon
adren/o	adrenal gland	colp/o	vagina
adrenal/o	adrenal gland	corne/o	cornea
aer/o	air	cost/o	ribs
albino/o	white	crani/o	cranium
angi/o	vessel	cutane/o	skin
an/o	anus	cyan/o	blue
append/o	appendix	cyt/o	cell
appendic/o	appendix	dent/o	teeth
aort/o	aorta	derm/o	skin
arteri/o	artery	dermat/o	skin
ather/o	thick, fatty	dipl/o	double
arthr/o	joint	duoden/o	duodenum
atri/o	atria	electr/o	electric
audi/o	hearing	encephal/o	brain
bacteri/o	bacteria	enter/o	small intestine
balan/o	glans penis	epiglott/o	epiglottis
blephar/o	eye lid	episi/o	vulva
bronch/o	bronchus	erethem/o	red
bronchi/o	bronchus	erythr/o	red
calc/o	calcium	esophag/o	esophagus
carcin/o	cancer	femor/o	femur
cardi/o	heart	fibul/o	fibula
carp/o	carpus	gastr/o	stomach
cerebr/o	brain	gli/o	glue, gluelike
cervic/o	cervix (neck)	glomerul/o	glomerulus
cholecyst/o	gallbladder	gloss/o	tongue

gluc/o	sugar	myring/o	eardrum
glyc/o	sugar	nas/o	nose
gynec/o	woman, female	nat/o	birth
hem/o	blood	necr/o	dead
hemat/o	blood	nephr/o	kidney
hepat/o	liver	neur/o	nerve
humer/o	humerus	noct/o	night
hydr/o	water	ocul/o	eye
hyster/o	uterus	olig/o	scanty
ile/o	ileum	onych/o	nail
jejun/o	jejunum	oophor/o	ovary
kerat/o	cornea, keratinized tissue	ophthalm/o	eye
lamin/o	lamina	or/o	mouth
lapar/o	abdomen	orch/o	testes
laryng/o	larynx	orchi/o	testes
leuk/o	white	orchid/o	testes
lingu/o	tongue	orth/o	straight
lip/o	fat	oste/o	bone
lith/o	stone	ot/o	ear
lumb/o	lumbar (low back)	ovari/o	ovary
lymph/o	lymph	ox/o	oxygen
mamm/o	breast	pancreat/o	pancreas
mast/o	breast	parathyroid/o	parathyroid
melan/o	black	patell/o	patella
men/o	menses	pelv/i	pelvis
mening/o	meninges	peritone/o	peritoneum
metacarp/o	metacarpus	phalang/o	phalanges
muc/o	mucus	pharyng/o	pharynx
myc/o	fungus	phleb/o	vein
myo	muscle	pil/o	hair
myel/o	spinal cord, bone marrow	pleur/o	pleura

(text continues on page 284)

pneum/o	lung, air	thorac/o	thorax
pneumon/o	lung, air	thromb/o	(clot) thrombus
proct/o	rectum, anus	thym/o	thymus
prostat/o	prostate	thyroid/o	thyroid
pulmon/o	lung	tibi/o	tibia
py/o	pus	tonsill/o	tonsil
pyel/o	renal pelvis	toxic/o	toxin, poison
rect/o	rectal	trache/o	trachea
ren/o	kidney	trich/o	hair
retin/o	retina	tympan/o	tympanic membrane
rhin/o	nose	ureter/o	ureter
salping/o	tubes (fallopian, eustachian)	urethr/o	urethra
scler/o	hardening	ur/o	urine
sigmoid/o	sigmoid colon	urin/o	urine
sinus/o	sinus	uter/o	uterus
sperm/o	sperm	vagin/o	vagina
spermat/o	sperm	vas/o	vessel
spin/o	spine	ven/o	vein
splen/o	spleen	ventricul/o	ventricle
stern/o	sternum	vertebr/o	vertebrae
stomat/o	mouth, mouthlike	vulv/o	vulva
ten/o	tendon	xanth/o	yellow
tend/o	tendon	xer/o	dry
tendin/o	tendon		

Term	Prefix	Combining Form	Suffix
abdomen		lapar/o	
abnormal condition			-osis
above, upon	epi-		
adrenal gland		adren/o, adrenal/o	
after, following	post-		
against	anti-		
air		aer/o	
anus		an/o	
around	circum-		
aorta		aort/o	
appendix		append/o, appendic/o	
artery		arteri/o	
atria		atri/o	
bacteria		bacteri/o	
bad, inadequate	mal-		
before, forward	pro-, pre-		
behind, back	re-, retro-		
below normal, beneath	hypo-, sub-		
between	inter-		
beyond	ultra-		
birth		nat/o	
black		melan/o	
blood		hemo, hemat/o	
blue		cyan/o	
bone		oste/o	
brain		cerebr/o, encephal/o	
breaking			-clasis, clast
breast		mamm/o, mast/o	
breathing			-pnea

(continues on page 286)

Term	Prefix	Combining Form	Suffix
bronchus		bronch/o, bronchi/o	
bursting forth			-rrhage, -rrhagia
calcium		calc/o	
cancer		carcin/o	
carpus		carp/o	
cartilage		chondr/o	
cell		cyt/o	-cyte
cervix		cervic/o	
cessation			-pause
clot		thromb/o	
colon		col/o, colon/o	
condition			-ia, -ism
condition of the blood			-emia
cornea		corne/o, kerat/o	
cranium		crani/o	
creating, producing			-gen, -genesis
crushing			-tripsy
cutting instrument			-tome
cutting into, incision			-tomy
dead		necr/o	
deficiency		olig/o	-penia
destroying, killing			-cide, -cidal
destruction of			-lysis
digestion			-pepsia
dilation, expansion			-ectasis
disease			-pathy
double		dipl/o	
drooping, prolapse			-ptosis
dry		xer/o	
duodenum		duoden/o	
ear		ot/o	

Term	Prefix	Combining Form	Suffix
eating, swallowing			-phage, -phagia
electric		electr/o	
enlargement			-megaly
epiglottis		epiglott/o	
esophagus		esophag/o	
excessive, above normal	supra-, hyper-		
excision, surgical removal			-ectomy
eye		ocul/o, ophthalm/o	
eyelid		blephar/o	
fat		adip/o, lip/o	
fear			-phobia
feeling			-phoria
femur		femor/o	
fibula		fibul/o	
flow, discharge			-rrhea
formation, growth			-plasia, -plasm
four	quadri-		
fungus		myc/o	
gallbladder		cholecyst/o	
gland		aden/o	
glans penis		balan/o	
glomerulus		glomerul/o	
glue, gluelike		gli/o	
good, normal	eu-		
hair		pil/o, trich/o	
half	hemi-		
hardening		scler/o	
hearing		audi/o	
heart		cardi/o	
hernia			-cele
humerus		humer/o	

(continues on page 288)

Term	Prefix	Combining Form	Suffix
ileum		ile/o	
inflammation			-itis
instrument for measuring			-meter
instrument to view			-scope
jejunum		jejun/o	
joint		arthr/o	
keratinized tissue, cornea		kerat/o, corne/o	
kidney		nephr/o, ren/o	
lamina		lamin/o	
large	macro-		
larynx		laryng/o	
liver		hepat/o	
lumbar		lumb/o	
lung		pulmon/o	
lymph		lymph/o	
lung, air		pneum/o, pneumon/o	
many, much	multi-, poly-		
measurement			-metry
menses		men/o	
meninges		mening/o, meningi/o	
metacarpus		metacarp/o	
mouth, mouthlike opening		or/o, stomat/o	-stomy
movement			-kinesia, -kinesis
mucus		muc/o	
muscle		my/o	
nail		onych/o	
narrowing, stricture			-stenosis
near, beside	peri-		
near, beside	para-		
nerve		neur/o	
new	neo-		

Term	Prefix	Combining Form	Suffix
night		noct/o	
nose		nas/o, rhin/o	
nourishment, growth			-trophy
one	uni-		
out, outside	ec-, ecto-		
ovary		oophor/o, ovari/o	
oxygen		ox/o	-oxia
pain			-algia, -dynia
painful, difficult	dys-		
pancreas		pancreat/o	
paralysis			-plegia
parathyroid		parathyroid/o	
patella		patell/o	
pathological condition or state			-iasis
pelvis		pelv/i	
peritoneum		peritone/o	
pertaining to			-ac, -al, -ar, -ary -eal, -(t)ic, -ical -ory, -(t)ous
phalanges		phalang/o	
pharynx		pharyng/o	
pleura		pleur/o	
poisonous, toxin	tox-	toxic/o	
positioned beneath	infra-		
pregnant woman			-gravida
process of recording			-graphy
prostate		prostat/o	
pus		py/o	
rapid	tachy-		
record			-gram
recording instrument			-graph

(continues on page 290)

Term	Prefix	Combining Form	Suffix
rectum		rect/o, proct/o	
red		erethem/o, erythr/o	
renal pelvis		pyel/o	
resembling			-oid
retina		retin/o	
ribs		cost/o	
rupture			-rrhexis
same, equal	iso-		
self	auto-		
sensation			-esthesia
sigmoid colon		sigmoid/o	
sinus		sinus/o	
skin		cutane/o, derm/o, dermat/o	-derma
slight or partial paralysis			-paresis
slow	brady-		
small	micro-		-ole, -ule
small intestine		enter/o	
softening			-malacia
specialist			-ist
specialist in the study of			-logist
speech			-phasia
sperm		sperm/o, spermat/o	
spine		spin/o	
spinal cord, bone marrow		myel/o	
spleen		splen/o	
sternum		stern/o	
stomach		gastr/o	
stone		lith/o	-lith
stopping			-stasis
straight		orth/o	
study of			-logy
sugar		gluc/o, glyc/o	

Term	Prefix	Combining Form	Suffix
surgical fixation			-pexy
surgical puncture			-centesis
surgical repair			-plasty
suture, suturing			-rrhaphy
swelling			-edema
teeth		dent/o	
tendon		ten/o, tend/o, tendin/o	
testes		orch/o, orchi/o, orchid/o, test/o	
thick, fatty		ather/o	
thirst			-dipsia
thorax		thorac/o	
three	tri-		
through, across	dia-, trans-		
thymus		thym/o	
thyroid		thyroid/o	
tibia		tibi/o	
tongue		gloss/o, lingu/o	
tonsil		tonsill/o	
toward	ad-		
trachea		trache/o	
treatment			-therapy
tubes		salping/o	
tumor			-oma
two	bi-		
tympanic membrane		tympan/o, myring/o	
ureter		ureter/o	
urethra		urethr/o	
urine		ur/o, urin/o	-uria
uterus		hyster/o, uter/o	
vagina		colp/o, vagin/o	
vein		phleb/o, ven/o	
ventricle		ventricul/o	

(continues on page 292)

Term	Prefix	Combining Form	Suffix
vertebrae		vertebr/o	
vessel		angi/o, vas/o	
vision			-opia
visual examination			-scopy
vomiting			-emesis
vulva		episi/o, vulv/o	
water		hydr/o	
white		albin/o, leuk/o	
within, inner	en-, endo-, intra-		
without, absence of	a-, an-, in-		
woman, female		gynec/o	
yellow		xanth/o	

GLOSSARY OF DIAGNOSTIC PROCEDURES

24-hour urine analysis: total urine excreted over a 24-hour period is collected for analysis

Arterial blood gases (ABGs): measures level of O_2, CO_2, and acid-base balance (pH) in arterial blood

Arthrogram: contrast medium is inserted into the joint space to outline soft-tissue structures; radiographs or MRI images are obtained; assesses persistent, unexplained joint pain

Audiometric tests: detailed hearing tests conducted by an audiologist

Barium enema: enema containing a substance that shows up well under x-ray and fluoroscopic examination

Barium swallow: x-ray examination of the esophagus during and after the patient swallows a liquid that contains barium

Biopsy: removal of a tissue sample for microscopic examination

Blood culture: whole blood is cultured to determine presence of infectious organisms and confirm diagnosis of sepsis

Blood urea nitrogen (BUN): laboratory value to measure kidney function based on nitrogen levels in the blood

Bone marrow aspiration: bone marrow specimen removed from cortex of a flat bone for analysis

Bone scan: gamma camera to detect abnormalities in bone density after injection of radioactive material

Bronchoscopy: provides direct visualization of the larynx, trachea, and bronchial tree with a bronchoscope for diagnostic and therapeutic reasons

Cardiac catheterization: evaluation of heart vessels and valves via injection of dye that shows up under radiology

Cerebrospinal fluid (CSF) analysis: analysis of fluid for blood, bacteria, or other abnormalities

Cholesterol, total: measurement of a lipid substance in the blood to determined risk of cardiovascular disease; desirable value is <200

Colonoscopy: visual inspection of the mucosa of the entire colon, ileocecal valve, and terminal ileum with a flexible fiberoptic colonoscope; used to determine cause of lower gastrointestinal disorders, remove foreign bodies and polyps, and stop bleeding

Complete blood count (CBC): key components of blood are measured and described; includes red blood cells (RBCs), white blood cells, (WBCs), hemoglobin, hematocrit level, platelets, and other components

Computed tomography (CT) scan: computerized collection and translation of multiple x-rays into a three-dimensional picture; creates a more detailed and accurate image than traditional x-rays

Continuous positive airway pressure (CPAP): device using positive air pressure to keep the airway open while a person sleeps; used for people with obstructive sleep apnea

Creatine kinase (CK): isoenzyme in skeletal and cardiac muscle released into the blood when muscle cells are damaged

Cryosurgery: destruction of abnormal tissue by freezing

Culture and sensitivity (C&S): growing microorganisms, then exposing them to antimicrobial drugs to determine which drugs kill them most effectively

D-dimer: test to help detect disseminated intravascular coagulation (DIC), deep vein thrombosis (DVT), myocardial infarction (MI), pulmonary embolism (PE), and unstable angina.

Dilation and curettage (D&C): cervix is dilated, then endometrial lining of uterus is scraped

Echocardiography: ultrasound procedure to detect cardiovascular disorders; allows visualization of the size, shape, position, thickness, and movement of all parts of the heart as well as characteristics of blood flow through the heart

Electroencephalography (EEG): records electrical activity of the brain on graph paper

Electromyogram (EMG): records electrical activity of skeletal muscles; diagnoses neuromuscular disorders

Endoscopic retrograde cholangiopan-creatography (ERCP): after a radiopaque material is injected though a fiber optic endoscope, radiographic examination of vessels that connect the liver, gallbladder, and pancreas to the duodenum

Enzyme-linked immunosorbent assay (ELISA): test for diagnosing HIV

Erythrocyte sedimentation rate (ESR), "sed" rate: rate at which red blood cells settle in a tube of unclotted blood; an elevated ESR indicates inflammation

Exercise stress test: noninvasive test that measures cardiac function during physical activity (treadmill test)

Fasting blood glucose (FBG): tests blood glucose levels after a 12-hour fast; screens for diabetes (fasting blood sugar [FBS])

Finger stick blood sugar (fsbs): blood glucose tested from a drop of capillary blood obtained by pricking the finger (finger stick blood glucose [fsbg])

Gastroccult: gastric contents are tested for the presence of blood and pH level

Glucose tolerance test (GTT): measures blood glucose levels at specified intervals after ingestion of glucose

Glycosylated hemoglobin (Hgb A1c): reflects average blood glucose level over the past 3–4 months

Hemoccult (stool guaiac test): small sample of feces tested for presence of blood

Holter monitor: records continuous heart activity for 24–48 hours; identifies arrhythmias and correlates them with any symptoms experienced by the patient

International normalized ratio (INR): standardized method of checking prothrombin time (PT), a blood clotting factor; monitors Coumadin therapy (Coumadin is a medication that slows clotting time)

Intravenous pyelogram (IVP): x-ray examination of the kidneys, ureters, and bladder after injection of a contrast medium

Laparoscopy: exploration of the contents of the abdomen by means of a laparo-scope

Lumbar puncture (LP): puncture of subarachnoid layer at 4th lumbar intervertebral space to obtain cerebrospinal fluid for analysis

Magnetic resonance imaging (MRI): uses an electromagnetic field and radio waves to create visual images on a computer screen

Mammography: x-ray examination to detect breast cancer

Needle biopsy: tissue or fluid is drawn through a large-gauge needle for analysis

Ova and parasites, stool: stool specimen is evaluated for presence of intestinal parasites (protozoa and worms) and their eggs

Papanicolaou's smear: cells are removed from the cervix and studied for cancer or other abnormalities

Partial thromboplastin time (PTT): measures blood clotting time; monitors heparin therapy (heparin is a medication that slows clotting time)

Patch test: a type of allergy test in which paper or gauze is saturated with an allergen and applied to the skin; test is positive if redness or swelling develops

Pelvic sonography: ultrasound imaging of structures in female pelvis

Prostate-specific antigen (PSA): blood test that screens for prostate cancer

Pulmonary angiography: radiographic examination of pulmonary circulation after injection of a contrast dye

Pulmonary function studies: tests that provide information about lung function, including volume, pattern, and rates of airflow

Pulse oximetry: indirect measure of arterial blood O_2 saturation level (SpO_2); normal level in a person with healthy lungs is 97%–99%

Rheumatoid factor: blood test to identify rheumatoid arthritis

Rinne's test: screening test for hearing; a comparison of bone conduction with air conduction by means of a tuning fork

Scratch test: allergy test in which allergens are scratched into the surface of the skin and the response is noted

Serum creatinine: laboratory value to measure kidney function; more specific value than BUN

Snellen eye chart: vision screening tool containing rows of letters in decreasing size

Sputum analysis: examination of mucus or fluid coughed up from the lungs

Stool culture: sample of feces examined for presence of bacteria and other microorganisms

Throat culture: tonsils and oropharynx swabbed for a specimen; specimen then cultured and tested for presence of bacterial organisms such as group A beta-hemolytic *Streptococci pyogenes*

Thyroid-stimulating hormone (TSH): reflects thyroid function; detects hypothyroidism

Tonometry: measurement of intraocular pressure

Transesophageal echocardiography (TEE): study of the heart via a probe placed in the esophagus

Transurethral resection of the prostate (TURP): removal of tissue from the prostate gland with an endoscope via the urethra

Triglycerides: fatty substance in the blood that contributes to the development of cardiovascular disease; desirable level in adults is <150

Troponin: most accurate blood test to confirm diagnosis of a myocardial infarction

Tubal ligation: sterilization procedure in which fallopian tubes are cut and ligated

Ultrasound: ultra-high frequency sound-waves outline shape of structures in the body

Upper endoscopy: visual examination of gastrointestinal tract from esophagus to duodenum

Urinalysis (UA): visual and microscopic analysis of a urine specimen

Vasectomy: sterilization procedure in which a small section of the vas deferens is removed

Vital capacity (VC): measurement of volume of air that can be exhaled after maximum inspiration

Weber's test: screening test for hearing; evaluates bone conduction using a tuning fork

MEDICAL TERMINOLOGY FAQs

Question: *How do I decide which word part to use when there is more than one to choose?*

Answer: It is often helpful to think of selecting the word part that is the most "user-friendly" to pronounce and that sounds best to the ear.

Example: Create a term that means "pertaining to the neck."

Choosing a combining form is easy because there is only one, *cervic/o*, which means *neck*. However, there are eight suffixes that mean "pertaining to." These are listed below with the selected combining form. Try pronouncing each version of the new term listed below. The first one is the easiest to pronounce and sounds best to the ear.

cervical
cervicac
cervicar
cervicary
cervicic
cervicical
cervicory
cerviceal

Question: *What if two options seem equally correct and desirable?*

Answer: Follow local custom.

Example: Create a term that means "pain in the neck."

There are two possible options: cervicalgia and cervicodynia. Either one is technically correct, so use the one that conforms to local custom. If you are unsure, make your best guess. The worst that will happen is that someone may be amused at your choice of terms. As you converse with and listen to your fellow healthcare professionals, you will quickly learn the preferred local terminology.

Question: *When a term includes more than one combining form, how do I know what order to put them in?*

Answer: If the term refers to a procedure, place the word parts in the order that corresponds with the procedure. If the term pertains to anatomy, move from most proximal to most distal.

Example: Create a term that means visual examination of the esophagus, stomach, and the duodenum.

As this procedure is performed, the scope first enters the esophagus, then the stomach, and then the duodenum. So when you create the medical term, put the word parts in the same order (with the suffix last): esophago-, gastro-, duodeno-, scopy.

Question: *I hear some terms pronounced in more than one way. How do I know which pronunciation is correct?*

Answer: First, refer to the pronunciation guide in this book. It should guide you in most cases. Second, in some cases more than one pronunciation may be considered acceptable. Third, remember that the most common mistake people make is to emphasize the wrong syllable. Remember that when word parts are linked with a combining vowel (usually the "o"), the emphasis is usually on the syllable with the combining vowel.

Example: The tendency is to pronounce colonoscopy as kō-lŏn-ō-SKŌ-pē. But the correct pronunciation is kō-lŏn-ŎS-kō-pē.

DRUGS AND DRUG CLASSIFICATIONS

There are several systems of drug classification. One is based on the body system that is most affected (e.g., respiratory drugs, cardiac drugs); another is based on the drug action (e.g., antihypertensive, antacid); another is based on the chemical action of the drug (e.g., cholinergic, selective serotonin reuptake inhibitor). As the following table indicates, most drugs fall into several different classes.

Drug (Trade/Generic Name)	Drug Classification	Common Use
Adrenaline/epinephrine	Adrenergic/bronchodilator/ vasopressor	Reversible airway obstruction caused by asthma, COPD, and anaphylaxis
Advil/ibuprofen Motrin/ibuprofen	NSAID/antipyretic/analgesic	Mild to moderate pain
Afrin/oxymetazoline	Local nasal decongestant	Nasal congestion
Aldactone/spironolactone	Potassium-sparing diuretic	Edema
Aleve/naproxen	NSAID/analgesic	Mild to moderate pain
Allegra/fexofenadine	Antihistamine	Seasonal allergies
Ambien/zolpidem	Miscellaneous sedative-hypnotic	Insomnia
Amoxil/amoxicillin	Penicillin/antibiotic	Infection
Asthmacort/triamcinolone acetonide	Inhalant corticosteroid	Asthma
Ativan/lorazapam	Benzodiazepine/antianxiety/sedative-hypnotic/anesthetic adjuvant/anticonvulsant	Anxiety, insomnia, preoperative sedation, status epilepticus
Atropine sulfate/atropine	Anticholinergic/antiarrhythmic	Bradycardia; given preoperatively to reduce oral secretions and bradycardia
Atrovent/ipratropium bromide	Anticholinergic bronchodilator	Asthma, COPD

(continues on page 300)

Drug (Trade/Generic Name)	Drug Classification	Common Use
Augmentin/amoxicillin, potassium clavulanate	Antibiotic/beta-lactimase inhibitor/aminopenicillin	Infection
Bayer aspirin/aspirin	NSAID/salicylate/analgesic/ antipyretic/platelet inhibitor	Mild to moderate pain, fever, prevention of thrombus formation
Bactrim/cotrimoxazole	Sulfonamide/antibiotic/antiprotozoal	Bacterial and protozoal infections
Benadryl/diphenhydramine HCl	Antihistamine/antiemetic/ anticholinergic	Allergies, nausea, minimizes some symptoms of Parkinson's disease
Bentyl/dicyclomine	Antispasmodic	Irritable bowel syndrome
Bumex/bumetanide	Loop diuretic/antihypertensive	Edema
Cardizem/diltiazem	Calcium ion antagonist (calcium chan-nel blocker)	Hypertension
Ceclor/cefaclor	Cephalosporin/antibiotic	Infection
Celebrex/celecoxib	NSAID, Cox-2 inhibitor	RA and OA
Cipro/ciprofloxacin	Fluoroquinolone/antibiotic	Infection
Codeine/codeine sulfate	Opiate agonist	Moderate to severe pain
Colace/docusate sodium	Fecal softener	Prevention or treatment of constipation
Compazine/prochlorperazine	Antiemetic/antipsychotic	Nausea, psychosis
Cordarone/amiodarone	Antiarrythymic	Arrhythmia
Coumadin/warfarin	Anticoagulant	Treats or prevents thrombus formation
Cozaar/losartan	Angiotensin II receptor blocker/ antihypertensive	Hypertension
Darvon/propoxyphene	Miscellaneous analgesic/opiate agonist	Mild to moderate pain
Decadron/dexamethasone	Corticosteroid/anti-inflammatory/ immunosuppressant	Cerebral edema
Deltasone/prednisone	Corticosteroid/anti-inflammatory	Allergies and inflammatory conditions
Demerol/meperidine	Opiate agonist	Moderate to severe pain
Detrol/tolterodine	Anticholinergic/urinary antispasmodic	Overactive bladder
Diabeta/glyburide	Oral hypoglycemic	NIDDM
Diflucan/fluconazole	Systemic antifungal	Fungal infection
Dilantin/phenytoin	Anticonvulsant	Seizure disorders
Dilaudid/hydromorphone	Opiate agonist	Moderate to severe pain
Ditropan/oxybutynin chloride	Urinary tract antispasmodic anticholinergic	Symptoms associated with neurogenic and overactive bladder

Drug (Trade/Generic Name)	Drug Classification	Common Use
Diuril/chlorothiazide	Thiazide diuretic/antihypertensive	HTN, CHF, edema
Dulcolax/bisacodyl	Laxative	Constipation
Dycil/dicloxacillin	Antibiotic/penicillinase-resistant penicillin	Infection
E-Mycin/erythromycin	Macrolide/antibiotic	Infection
Elavil/amitriptyline	Tricyclic antidepressant	Depression
Eskalith/lithium	Antimanic	Bipolar disorder
Flagyl/metronidazole	Miscellaneous anti-infective	Bacterial, fungal or protozoal infection
Flexeril/cyclobenzaprine	Centrally acting skeletal muscle relaxant	Muscle spasm associated with painful musculoskeletal conditions
Flonase/fluticasone	Intranasal corticosteroid	Allergies, asthma
Fosamax/alendronate	Bone resorption inhibitor/ biphosphonate	Prevention and treatment of osteoporosis
Glucophage/metformin	Biguanide oral hypoglycemic	NIDDM
Heparin sodium/heparin	Anticoagulant	Prevention and treatment of thrombus, MI, and PE
Hytrin/terazosin	α-1 adrenergic blocker/ antihypertensive	Hypertension, BPH
Imodium/loperamide	Antidiarrheal	Diarrhea
Isopto Carpine/pilocarpine	Direct acting cholinergic	Open angle glaucoma
Lanoxin/digoxin	Digitalis glycoside/antiarrhythmic/cardiotonic/inotropic	Atrial arrhythmias; CHF
Lopressor/metoprolol	β-adrenergic blocker (β blocker)/antihypertensive/antianginal/antiarrythmic	Hypertension, MI, angina, arrhythmias
Lasix/furosemide	Loop diuretic	Edema, CHF, HTN, heart failure
Lipitor/atorvastatin	Antihyperlipedemic	Hypercholesterolemia, hyperlipedemia
Lomotil/diphenoxylate with atropine	Antidiarrheal	Diarrhea
Lovenox/enoxaparin	Anticoagulant	Treatment or prevention of DVT
Luminal/phenobarbital	Barbiturate/sedative-hypnotic/antiseizure	Seizure disorders; given as preoperative sedation
Lunesta/eszopiclone	Nonbenzodiazepine hypnotic	Insomnia
Macrodantin/nitrofurantoin	Quinolone/miscellaneous anti-infective	UTI
Metamucil/psyllium hydrophilic mucilloid	Bulk-forming laxative	Prevention or treatment of constipation, IBS

(continues on page 302)

Drug (Trade/Generic Name)	Drug Classification	Common Use
Monistat 3/miconazole	Topical antifungal	Various fungal infections
MS Contin/morphine	Opiate agonist	Moderate to severe pain
Mucomyst/acetylcysteine	Mucolytic	Liquefies thick mucus
Naproxen/Aleve	NSAID	Mild to moderate pain
Narcan/naloxone	Opiate antagonist	Reverses effects of opiate agonists and opiate partial agonists (given for overdoses)
Neurontin/gabapentin	Miscellaneous anticonvulsant	Seizure disorders, neuropathic pain
Niacin/nicotinic acid	Antihyperlipidemic/vitamin	High LDL, VLDL, and cholesterol
Nitrostat/nitroglycerine	Nitrate/antianginal	Angina, HTN, MI
Oxycontin/oxycodone	Opiate agonist	Moderate to severe pain
Paxil/paroxetine	Antidepressant/antianxiety	Depression, panic disorder, OCD, generalized anxiety disorder
Pepcid/famotidine	Histamine (H2) receptor antagonist	GERD, ulcers
Persantine/dipyridamole	Platelet inhibitor	MI, TIA, stroke, thrombotic disorders
Phenergan/promethazine	Antihistamine/antiemetic/sedative-hypnotic	Nausea
Premarin/conjugated estrogen	Estrogen	Menopause
Procardia/nifedipine	Calcium ion antagonist (calcium channel blocker)/antihypertensive	Hypertension
Protonix/pantoprazole	Gastric acid pump inhibitor/antiulcer	GERD, ulcers
Proventil/albuterol	Adrenergic/bronchodilator	Asthma, COPD
Provera/medroxyprogesterone	Progestin	Amenorrhea, abnormal uterine bleeding
Prozac/fluoxetine	Antidepressant/SSRI	Depression
Pyridium/phenazopyridine HCl	Nonopiate urinary tract analgesic	Pain caused by UTI
Quinaglute/quinidine	Antiarrhythmic	Arrhythmia
Reglan/metoclopramide	Prokinetic/antiemetic	Nausea, esophagitis, GERD
Retrovir (AZT)/zidovudine	Antiviral	HIV/AIDS
Risperdal/risperidone	Antipsychotic	Psychotic disorders, dementia-related psychotic symptoms
Ritalin/methylphenidate	CNS stimulant	ADHD, narcolepsy

Drug (Trade/Generic Name)	Drug Classification	Common Use
Robaxin/methocarbamol	Centrally acting skeletal muscle relaxant	Muscle spasm associated with acute painful musculoskeletal conditions
Robitussin/guaifenesin	Expectorant	Thick respiratory secretions
Rocephin/ceftriaxone	Cephalosporin (antibiotic)	Infection
Roxicodone/oxycodone	Opiate agonist	Moderate to severe pain
Sinemet/carbidopa, levodopa	Antiparkinsonian/dopamine agonist	Parkinson's disease
Singulair/montelukast	Antileukotriene	Asthma
Solumedrol/methylpred-nisolone	Corticosteroid/anti-inflammatory, immunosuppressant	Inflammatory disorders, numerous chronic diseases
Stadol/butorphanol	Opiate partial agonist	Moderate to severe pain
Straterra/atomoxetine	SNRI	ADHD
Streptomycin/streptomycin	Aminoglycoside/antibiotic	Infection
Sudafed/pseudoephedrine	Decongestant	Nasal congestion, rhinitis
Symmetrel/amantadine HCl	Antiviral/antiparkinsonian	Parkinson's disease, influenza A
Synthroid/levothyroxine	Thyroid hormone	Hypothyroidism
Tegretol/carbamazepine	Miscellaneous anticonvulsant	Seizure disorders, neuropathic pain
Tequin/gatifloxacin	Fluoroquinolone/antibiotic	Infection
Timoptic/timolol maleate	β-adrenergic blocker	Open-angle glaucoma, ocular HTN
Toradol/ketorolac	NSAID/analgesic	Mild to moderate pain
Trental/pentoxifylline	Hemorrheologic	Intermittent claudication caused by peripheral vascular disease
TUMS/calcium carbonate	Antacid	GERD
Tylenol/acetaminophen	Miscellaneous analgesic/antipyretic	Mild to moderate pain, fever
Ultram/tramadol	Opiate agonist	Moderate pain
Valium/diazepam	Benzodiazepine/antianxiety/sedative-hypnotic/antiseizure/skeletal muscle relaxant	Anxiety, given as preoperative sedation, status epilepticus, skeletal muscle spasm
Vasotec/enalapril	ACE inhibitor/antihypertensive	Hypertension
Versed/midazolam	Benzodiazepine/antianxiety/sedative-hypnotic	Preoperative sedation, conscious sedation
Viagra/sildenafil	Phosphodiesterase inhibitor	Erectile dysfunction
Vibramycin/doxycycline	Tetracycline/antibiotic	Infection
Wellbutrin/bupropion	Antidepressant/smoking deterrant	Depression, smoking cessation

(continues on page 304)

Drug (Trade/Generic Name)	Drug Classification	Common Use
Xanax/alprazolam	Benzodiazepine/anxiolytic	Anxiety, panic disorders
Xylocaine/lidocaine	Antiarrhythmic/local anesthetic	Arrhythmias, local anesthesia for suturing
Zantac/ranitidine	Histamine-2 blocker	GERD, PUD
Zithromax/azithromycin	Macrolide/antibiotic	Infection
Zocor/simvastatin	Antihyperlipedemic/HCG-COA reductase inhibitor	High cholesterol and LDL
Zofran/ondansetron	Antiemetic	Nausea
Zoloft/xertraline	SSRI/antidepressant	Depression, obsessive-compulsive disorder
Zovirax/acyclovir	Antiviral	Oral and genital herpes
Zyprexa/olanzepline	Atypical antipsychotic	Psychotic disorders, dementia-related psychotic symptoms

Analgesic Combination Products

Darvocet-N 100	Acetaminophen, 650 mg	Propoxyphene napsylate, 100 mg
Percocet	Acetaminophen, 500 mg	Oxycodone, 5 mg
Tylenol #3	Acetaminophen, 325 mg	Codeine, 30 mg

For a list of the most commonly prescribed drugs, see www.rxlist.com

ANSWERS TO CHAPTER EXERCISES

G

CHAPTER 1

Matching
Exercise A
1. f
2. i
3. j
4. b
5. g
6. g
7. d
8. c
9. e
10. a

Exercise B
1. d
2. e
3. g
4. b
5. h
6. i
7. j
8. c
9. f
10. a

True or False
1. True
2. True

3. True
4. True

Fill in the Blank
1. uni
2. quadri
3. micro
4. para & peri
5. poly & multi

SUFFIXES
Matching
Exercise A
1. f
2. h
3. g
4. a
5. h
6. j
7. c
8. i
9. e
10. i

Exercise B
1. i
2. d
3. f
4. c
5. a

6. g
7. k
8. g
9. j
10. h
11. b

True or False
1. True
2. False
3. False
4. False
5. True
6. False
7. False
8. True
9. True
10. False
11. True
12. False

Fill in the Blank
1. -kinesia & -kinesis
2. -gram
3. -paresis
4. -stomy
5. -oma
6. -plegia
7. -ptosis

8. -stasis & -pause
9. -stenosis
10. -lith
11. -centesis
12. -ectasis
13. -al, -ac, -ar, -ary, -ia, -(t)ic, -ical, -ory, -eal, -(t)ous

Multiple Choice

1. a
2. d
3. c
4. c
5. b

Deciphering Terms

1. pertaining to two sides
2. flow through
3. pertaining to poison
4. pertaining to one side
5. a condition of below normal oxygen
6. large eating (name of a type of white blood cell that "eats" bacteria)
7. forward movement
8. self-recording instrument
9. paralysis of two (legs)
10. paralysis of four (extremities)
11. painful or difficult (bad) feeling
12. good feeling
13. many fears

CHAPTER 2

Matching
Exercise A

1. e
2. j
3. j
4. d
5. g
6. a
7. h
8. e
9. j
10. b

Exercise B

1. k
2. f
3. b
4. i
5. a
6. h
7. d
8. f
9. j
10. i
11. a

Word Building

1. adipoid, lipoid
2. xerodermal
3. albinism, leukism
4. xanthosis
5. dermal
6. epidermal
7. dermatomycosis, dermomycosis
8. erythrocytopenia
9. circumoral cyanosis
10. scleroderma, dermosclerosis
11. trichomycosis
12. keratosis
13. leukemia
14. onycomycosis
15. melanoma
16. necrosis, necrotic
17. hypodermic
18. lipectomy, adipectomy
19. adipocyte, lipocyte
20. xeroderma

Deciphering Terms

1. blue skin
2. pertaining to hardness
3. abnormal condition of excessive keratinized tissue
4. deficiency of white (blood) cells
5. pertaining to beneath the skin
6. red (blood) cell
7. study of the skin
8. black cell
9. abnormal condition of hair fungus
10. excessive nourishment or growth
11. dry skin
12. yellow tumor
13. destruction of fat
14. abnormal condition of fat
15. nail tumor
16. abnormal condition of death (dead tissue)

True or False

1. True
2. False
3. True
4. True
5. False
6. False
7. False
8. True
9. True
10. False
11. True

Fill in the Blank

1. abrasion
2. ecchymosis, contusion
3. petechia
4. impetigo
5. vitiligo
6. vesicle
7. pustule
8. comedo
9. scabies
10. papule
11. alopecia
12. laceration
13. fissure
14. eczema
15. macule
16. cellulitis
17. tinea
18. scales
19. cyst

Common Diagnostic Tests

1. **Patch allergy test:** paper or gauze saturated with an allergen is applied to the skin; the test is positive if redness or swelling develops

2. **Scratch allergy test:** allergens are scratched into the surface of the skin, and the response is noted

3. **Biopsy**: removal of a tissue sample for microscopic examination

Multiple Choice

1. b
2. d
3. c
4. d
5. c

Case Study Questions

1. b
2. a
3. c
4. a
5. d
6. d
7. a
8. b
9. c
10. d

CHAPTER 3

Matching

1. g
2. e
3. f
4. a
5. a
6. b
7. d

Word Building

1. polyneuritis
2. infraspinous, infraspinal
3. myelomeningocele
4. encephalomeningitis
5. paraspinal, paraspinous
6. glioma
7. isoelectric
8. hemiparesis
9. quadriplegia
10. paraplegia
11. encephalopathy
12. neuralgia

Deciphering Terms

1. pertaining to the brain and spine
2. disease of the nerves
3. tumor of spinal cord or bone marrow
4. inflammation of the meninges
5. process of recording brain (activity)
6. glue cell
7. abnormal condition of brain hardening
8. paralysis of half (of the body)
9. pertaining to paralysis of two (legs)
10. partial paralysis of four (extremities)
11. inflammation of nerves

True or False

1. False
2. True
3. True
4. True
5. False
6. True
7. True
8. True
9. True
10. False

Fill in the Blank

1. epilepsy
2. Bell's palsy
3. cerebrovascular accident (CVA)
4. spina bifida
5. transient ischemic attack (TIA)
6. Huntington's chorea

Common Diagnostic Tests

1. **Cerebrospinal fluid (CSF) analysis:** analysis of fluid for blood, bacteria, or other abnormalities
2. **Computed tomography (CT):** study of brain and spinal cord using radiology and computer analysis
3. **Electroen-cephalography (EEG):** records electrical activity of the brain
4. **Electromyogram (EMG):** record of muscle activity as a result of electrical stimulation
5. **Lumbar puncture (LP):** puncture of subarach-noid space at 4th intervertebral space to obtain CSF fluid for analysis
6. **Magnetic resonance imaging (MRI):** uses an electromagnetic field and radio waves to create visual images on a computer screen

Multiple Choice

1. d
2. c
3. a
4. d
5. b

Case Study Questions

1. a
2. c
3. b
4. a
5. b
6. b
7. false

CHAPTER 4

Matching
Exercise A

1. h
2. e
3. d
4. f
5. i
6. b
7. c
8. i
9. a

Exercise B

1. e
2. g
3. h
4. a
5. b
6. c
7. h
8. d

Word Building

1. angiogram, vasogram
2. aortic
3. arteriography
4. atherosclerosis
5. atriorrhexis
6. bradycardia
7. cardiomegaly
8. tachycardia
9. electrocardiogram
10. hematologist
11. lymphoid
12. phlebotomy
13. splenomegaly
14. thrombocyte
15. angioplasty, vasoplasty
16. ventriculocele
17. adenopathy
18. microcardia

Deciphering Terms

1. a condition of a small heart
2. a small vein
3. a record of blood
4. process of recording a vessel
5. surgical repair of the aorta
6. a small artery
7. thick, fatty cell
8. pain in the atrium
9. pertaining to electricity
10. blood in the urine
11. disease of the lymph glands
12. inflammation of a vein
13. stopping a vein (refers to sluggish blood flow)
14. softening of the spleen
15. destruction of a clot
16. pain in a vessel
17. surgical repair of the ventricle

True or False

1. False
2. True
3. True
4. True
5. False
6. False
7. True
8. False
9. False
10. True
11. True
12. True

Fill in the Blank

1. arrhythmia
2. transient ischemic attack, TIA
3. bruit
4. 3 times a day
5. congestive heart failure
6. each evening
7. deep vein thrombosis, DVT
8. partial thromboplastin time, PTT
9. every 2 hours
10. myocardial infarction, MI
11. varicose veins
12. lymphatic cancer
13. RA & LA
14. RV & LV
15. CAD
16. blood pressure, hypertension
17. electrocardiogram
18. four
19. acquired immuno-deficiency syndrome
20. human immuno-deficiency, HIV
21. *Pneumocystis carinii* pneumonia
22. twice a day
23. each morning
24. stroke, CVA, or brain attack

Common Diagnostic Tests

Cardiovascular System

1. **Cardiac catheteriza-tion:** evaluation of heart vessels and valves via the injection of dye that shows up under radiology
2. **International norma-lized ratio (INR):** standardized method of checking the pro-thrombin time (PT), a blood clotting factor, used to monitor Coumadin therapy
3. **Partial thromboplastin time (PTT):** measures blood clotting time, used to determine therapeutic level of heparin
4. **Transesophageal echocardiography (TEE):** a study of the heart via a probe placed in the esophagus
5. **Troponin:** most accurate blood test to confirm diagnosis of MI

Lymphatic/Immune Systems

1. **Enzyme-linked immunosorbent assay (ELISA):** test for diagnosing HIV
2. **Erythrocyte sedimentation rate (ESR):** test that indicates inflammation in the body

Multiple Choice

1. d
2. a
3. c
4. a
5. b

Case Study Questions

1. b
2. a
3. d
4. b
5. b
6. c
7. c
8. b
9. d

CHAPTER 5

Matching
Exercise A

1. i
2. b
3. e
4. d
5. h
6. a
7. i
8. c
9. a

Exercise B

1. f
2. b
3. j
4. h
5. c
6. d
7. i
8. g
9. a
10. e

Word Building

1. bronchopulmonary
2. chondroma
3. aerogenesis
4. mucocutaneous
5. tracheobronchoscopy
6. tonsillopathy
7. tracheomalacia
8. epiglottitis
9. perinasal
10. dyspneic
11. eupnea
12. thoracotomy
13. pharyngomycosis
14. pleurodynia
15. pneumopexy, pulmonopexy
16. pulmonary, pulmonic
17. sinusoid
18. tracheostomy
19. carcinogenic
20. tachypnea
21. laryngoscopy

Deciphering Terms

1. pertaining to the larynx
2. pain in the pleura
3. pertaining to air or lungs
4. a condition of the lungs
5. pertaining to the lungs
6. incision into the sinus
7. surgical puncture of the thorax
8. surgical removal of the tonsils
9. painful or difficult breathing
10. blood in the thorax (pleural space)
11. air in the thorax (pleural space)
12. good or normal breathing
13. breathing in a straight (upright) position
14. inflammation of the nose
15. mouthlike opening in the trachea
16. swallowing air
17. pertaining to the pharynx
18. pertaining to the nose
19. destruction of mucus
20. cancerous tumor

True or False

1. False
2. True
3. True
4. False
5. False
6. True
7. False
8. True
9. True
10. False
11. False
12. True
13. True
14. True
15. False
16. True
17. True
18. False
19. False
20. True

Fill in the Blank

1. chronic obstructive pulmonary disease
2. COPD
3. asthma
4. coryza
5. pneumothorax
6. stridor
7. stat
8. upper respiratory infection
9. cardiopulmonary resuscitation (CPR)
10. nosebleed

Common Diagnostic Tests

1. **Vital capacity (VC):** measurement of volume of air that can be exhaled after maximum inspiration
2. **Pulmonary angiography:** radiographic examination of pulmonary circulation after injection of a contrast dye
3. **Arterial blood gases (ABGs):** measure level of O_2, CO_2 and acid-base balance (pH) in arterial blood
4. **Pulse oximetry:** indirect measurement of arterial blood O_2, saturation level
5. **Sputum analysis:** examines sample of mucus or fluid coughed up from the lungs

Multiple Choice

1. c
2. a
3. b
4. c
5. a

Case Study Questions

1. b
2. d
3. a
4. b
5. d
6. d
7. b

CHAPTER 6

Matching
Exercise A

1. f
2. i
3. h
4. b
5. a
6. j
7. f
8. e
9. a
10. d

Exercise B

1. d
2. f
3. h
4. j
5. a

6. e
7. b
8. i
9. g
10. d

Word Building

1. hepatopathy
2. esophagitis
3. esophagogastroscopy
4. circumoral
5. cholecystectomy
6. gastromegaly
7. hypercolonic
8. perianal
9. jejunostomy
10. hepatoma
11. appendicitis
12. appendectomy
13. iliotomy
14. hyperemesis
15. dental
16. cholecystitis
17. hypogastric
18. colonoscopy
19. cholelith
20. colonopathy

Deciphering Terms

1. excision or surgical removal of the gallbladder
2. inflammation of the small intestine
3. visual examination of the anus and rectum
4. instrument used to view the stomach

5. visual examination of the abdomen

6. surgical repair of the jejunum

7. a stone in the pancreas

8. pertaining to beneath or under the tongue

9. inflammation of the pharynx (sore throat)

10. specialist in the study of the stomach and (small) intestines

11. pertaining to a small stomach

12. painful or difficult movement

13. to flow through (passage of frequent loose stools)

14. partial paralysis of the stomach

15. painful or difficult feeling (a bad or depressed mood)

16. absence of nourishment or growth

17. the study (of disorders) of the rectum and anus

18. crushing of a stone

19. painful or difficult digestion (upset stomach or heartburn)

20. mouth pain

True or False

1. False
2. True
3. False
4. True
5. True
6. True
7. False
8. False
9. False
10. True
11. True
12. False
13. True
14. True
15. False
16. True
17. False
18. True
19. True

Fill in the Blank

1. ascites
2. diverticulosis
3. diverticulitis
4. endoscopic retrograde cholangiopancreatography
5. emesis
6. $\bar{c}$
7. ulcerative colitis
8. Abd
9. upper gastrointestinal
10. small bowel obstruction
11. NPO
12. PO
13. PR
14. VS qh
15. qd
16. intussusception
17. jaundice
18. CA
19. BR $\bar{c}$ BRP
20. complained of nausea and vomiting

Common Diagnostic Tests

1. **Barium enema:** enema containing a substance that shows up well under x-ray and fluoroscopic examination

2. **Barium swallow:** x-ray examination of the esophagus while and after the patient swallows a liquid that contains barium; abnormalities of the esophagus may be seen

3. **Computed tomography (CT) scan:** computerized collection and translation of multiple x-rays into a three-dimensional picture; creates a more detailed and accurate image than does traditional x-rays

4. **Endoscopic retrograde cholangiopancreatography (ERCP):** radiographic examination of vessels that connect the liver, gallbladder, and pancreas to the duodenum after a radiopaque material is injected though a fiberoptic endoscope

5. **Gastroccult:** gastric contents are tested for the presence of blood and pH level

6. **Hemoccult (stool guaiac test):** small sample of feces is tested for presence of blood

7. **Laparoscopy:** exploration of the contents of the abdomen using a laparoscope

8. **Lower endoscopy:** visual examination of the GI tract, from rectum to cecum

9. **Stool culture:** sample of the feces is examined for presence of bacteria and other microorganisms

10. **Ultrasound:** ultra-high frequency soundwaves are used to outline the shape of various structures in the body

11. **Upper endoscopy:** visual examination of the GI tract, from esophagus to duodenum

Multiple Choice

1. c
2. b
3. c
4. a
5. c
6. b

Case Study Questions

1. d
2. c
3. b
4. a
5. b
6. d
7. a

CHAPTER 7

Matching
Exercise A

1. d
2. a
3. i
4. f
5. g
6. c
7. h
8. b
9. c

Exercise B

1. a
2. i
3. f
4. h
5. g
6. f
7. c
8. b
9. h

Word Building

1. anuria
2. polyuria
3. pyuria
4. dysuria
5. oliguric
6. urethrodynia, urethralgia
7. cystoscopy
8. hematuria
9. nephrolithiasis
10. nocturia
11. bacteremia
12. ureterectomy
13. pyelonephritis
14. urethrocystogram
15. urinal, uric
16. glycogenesis
17. renal
18. glomerulonephritis
19. antibacterial
20. hemolysis

Deciphering Terms

1. disease of the kidney
2. surgical fixation of the urethra
3. beside or near the urethra
4. excision or surgical removal of the bladder
5. incision into the kidney
6. mouthlike opening in the ureter
7. inflammation of the glomerulus and kidney
8. much thirst
9. excision or surgical removal of the kidney
10. urination at night
11. bacteria in the urine
12. blood in the urine
13. kidney stone
14. pertaining to absence of urination
15. enlargement of the bladder
16. pertaining to behind the peritoneum

True or False

1. True
2. False
3. False
4. True
5. False
6. False
7. True
8. True
9. True
10. True

Fill in the Blank

1. glycosuria, glucosuria
2. ESRD
3. UTI
4. enuresis
5. phimosis
6. uremia
7. diuresis
8. interstitial cystitis
9. interstitial nephritis
10. pyelonephritis
11. urinary retention
12. stress incontinence

Common Diagnostic Tests

1. **Blood urea nitrogen (BUN):** laboratory value used to measure kidney function based on nitrogen levels in the blood
2. **Culture and sensitivity (C&S):** growing microorganisms, then exposing them to antimicrobial drugs to determine which ones kill them most effectively
3. **24-hour urine specimen:** total urine excreted over a 24-hour period is collected for analysis
4. **Intravenous pyelogram (IVP):** x-ray examination of the kidneys, ureters, and bladder after injection of a contrast medium
5. **Serum creatinine:** laboratory value used to measure kidney function; more specific than BUN
6. **Urinalysis (UA):** visual and microscopic analysis of urine

Multiple Choice

1. c
2. d
3. b
4. b
5. c

Case Study Questions

1. d
2. c
3. b
4. c
5. a
6. b
7. d
8. a
9. c

CHAPTER 8

Matching
Exercise A

1. c
2. g
3. j
4. h
5. c
6. i
7. c
8. f
9. c
10. f
11. a
12. k
13. h

Exercise B

1. e
2. g
3. b
4. a
5. f
6. h
7. j
8. j
9. f
10. h
11. k
12. k

Word Building

1. balanitis
2. episiotomy
3. anorchidism
4. orchidopexy
5. oligospermia

6. perinatal
7. dysplasia
8. neoplasia, neoplasm
9. retrovaginal
10. anesthesia
11. vasostenosis
12. prostatodynia, prostatalgia
13. cervicitis
14. vaginorrhaphy, colporrhaphy
15. gynecologist
16. laparoscope
17. hysterectomy
18. mammogram
19. mastopexy, mammopexy
20. menopause
21. multigravida
22. oophoroma
23. colpocele, vaginocele
24. salpingorrhexis

Deciphering Terms

1. gynecology
2. noncancerous uterine tumors
3. oral contraceptives
4. a fertilized ovum is implanted outside of the uterus
5. transurethral resection of the prostate
6. proliferation of endometrial tissue in the abdominopelvic area
7. total abdominal hysterectomy, bilateral salpingo-oophorectomy

8. a sexually transmitted disease caused by an infestation with parasite genus *Trichomonas*, which causes vaginitis, urethritis, and cystitis
9. dilation or expansion of the testes
10. surgical excision of one or both of the ovaries and fallopian tubes
11. surgical repair of the glans penis
12. painful or difficult (abnormal) cell/tissue growth
13. pertaining to new cell/tissue growth
14. process of recording the breasts
15. visual examination of the abdomen
16. suturing of the testes
17. many pregnancies
18. cessation of menses
19. excessive cell/tissue growth
20. herniation of the prostate

True or False

1. True
2. False
3. True
4. False
5. False
6. True
7. True
8. True
9. False
10. False
11. True
12. False
13. True
14. False
15. True

Fill in the Blank

1. ectopic
2. endometriosis
3. syphilis
4. total abdominal hysterectomy, fibroids
5. obstetrician-gynecologist
6. trichomoniasis
7. oral contraceptive
8. Papanicolaou's smear
9. sterility
10. in vitro fertilization
11. total abdominal hysterectomy, bilateral salpingo-oophorectomy
12. benign prostatic hypertrophy
13. transurethral resection of the prostate
14. impotence

Common Diagnostic Tests

1. **Cryosurgery:** destruction of abnormal tissue by freezing
2. **Dilation and curettage (D&C):** cervix is dilated and endometrial lining of uterus is scraped
3. **Needle biopsy:** tissue or fluid is drawn through a large-gauge needle for analysis

4. **Papanicolaou's smear:** cells are removed from the cervix and studied for cancer or other abnormalities
5. **Pelvic sonography:** ultrasound imaging of structures in female pelvis
6. **Prostate-specific antigen (PSA):** blood test used to screen for prostate cancer
7. **Transurethral resection of the prostate (TURP):** removal of tissue from the prostate gland with an endoscope via the urethra
8. **Tubal ligation:** sterilization procedure in which fallopian tubes are cut and ligated
9. **Vasectomy:** sterilization procedure in which a small section of the vas deferens is removed

Multiple Choice
1. c
2. a
3. c
4. a
5. d

Case Study Questions
1. a
2. c
3. c
4. d
5. c

6. d
7. a

CHAPTER 9

Exercise A
1. h
2. g
3. i
4. g
5. c
6. g
7. b
8. g
9. a

Exercise B
1. e
2. g
3. b
4. a
5. d
6. g
7. d
8. c
9. c

Word Building
1. toxicologist
2. adenoma
3. hypoparathyroid
4. adrenalopathy
5. hypercalcemia
6. glucometer
7. hydrotherapy
8. oophorocentesis
9. anorchism
10. pancreatitis

11. euthymic
12. hyperthyroidism

Deciphering Terms
1. pertaining to the pancreas
2. herniation of the ovary
3. pain of the testes
4. disease of the adrenal (gland)
5. suturing of the testes
6. normal blood sugar
7. pertaining to painful or difficult (abnormal) thymus
8. rupture of the thyroid
9. disease of a gland
10. deficiency of sugar
11. a condition of low blood sugar

True or False
1. True
2. False
3. False
4. True
5. False
6. False
7. False
8. True
9. True
10. True
11. False

Fill in the Blank
1. blood sugar
2. dwarfism
3. cancer
4. calcium
5. T3 and T4

6. DM

7. noninsulin-dependent diabetes mellitus

8. insulin-dependent diabetes mellitus

9. growth hormone

10. exophthalmos

11. gigantism

12. Graves' disease

13. Cushing's syndrome

14. myxedema

15. Addison's

16. cretinism

Common Diagnostic Tests

1. **fasting blood glucose (FBG):** fasting blood sugar (FBS); tests blood glucose levels after a 12-hour fast; used to screen for diabetes

2. **finger stick blood sugar (fsbs):** finger stick blood glucose (fsbg); blood glucose tested from a drop of capillary blood obtained by pricking the finger

3. **glucose tolerance test (GTT):** measures blood glucose levels at specified intervals after ingestion of glucose

4. **glycosylated hemoglobin (Hgb A1c):** reflects average blood glucose level over the past 3-4 months

5. **thyroid stimulating hormone (TSH):** reflects thyroid function; detects hypothyroidism

Multiple Choice

1. c
2. c
3. b
4. c
5. a

Case Study Questions

1. c
2. a
3. d
4. b

CHAPTER 10

Matching
Exercise A

1. g
2. m
3. f
4. i
5. d
6. b
7. c
8. h
9. j
10. k
11. a
12. e

Exercise B

1. j
2. d
3. f
4. h
5. l
6. b
7. l

8. c
9. e
10. l
11. i
12. k
13. a

Word Building

1. costovertebral
2. osteoarthritis
3. carpal
4. paracervical
5. chondrodynia, chondralgia
6. laminotome
7. intercostal
8. cranioplasty
9. femoral
10. humeral
11. orthopnea
12. lumbodynia, lumbalgia
13. metacarpitis
14. myeloma
15. myoplegia
16. substernal
17. osteopathy
18. patellectomy
19. pelvimetry
20. phalangitis
21. tendinitis
22. thoracolumbar
23. tibiomalacia
24. vertebroplasty

Deciphering Terms

1. beside or near the vertebra

2. pertaining to above the tibia

3. pertaining to the thorax

4. destruction of a tendon

5. incision into the sternum

6. pertaining to the phalanges

7. drooping of the patella

8. incision into the bone

9. disease of the muscle

10. abnormal condition of hardening of the bone marrow or spinal cord

11. pertaining to the lower back

12. incision into the lamina (a portion of a vertebra)

13. pain in the femur

14. incision into the cranium

15. inflammation of the ribs and cartilage

16. inflammation of the neck (or cervix)

17. surgical puncture of the carpus

18. pain in a joint

19. breaking of a bone

20. pertaining to outside of the tibia

True or False

1. False

2. True

3. False

4. True

5. True

6. True

7. True

8. False

9. True

10. False

Fill in the Blank

1. below the knee amputation, BKA

2. scoliosis

3. osteoarthritis

4. strain

5. osteoarthritis

6. C1-C7

7. crepitus

8. carpal tunnel syndrome

9. CTS

10. total knee replacement, total hip replacement

11. S1-S5

12. straight or upright

13. fracture, Fx

14. anteroposterior, AP

15. L1-L5

16. herniated disk

17. T1-T12

18. rheumatoid

19. above the knee amputation, AKA

Common Diagnostic Tests

1. **Bone marrow aspiration:** bone marrow specimen is removed from cortex of a flat bone for analysis

2. **Bone scan:** a gamma camera is used to detect abnormalities in bone density after injection of radioactive material

3. **Creatine kinase (CK):** isoenzyme in skeletal and cardiac muscle released into the blood when muscle cells are damaged

4. **Electromyogram (EMG):** records electrical activity of skeletal muscles; used to diagnose neuromuscular disorders

5. **Erythrocyte sedimentation rate (ESR) or "sed" rate:** rate at which red blood cells settle in a tube of unclotted blood; elevated ESR indicates inflammation

6. **Rheumatoid factor:** blood test used to identify rheumatoid arthritis

Multiple Choice

1. d

2. a

3. a

4. a

5. d

Case Study Questions

1. d

2. b

3. a

4. c

CHAPTER 11

Matching

Exercise A

1. e
2. b
3. a
4. a
5. d
6. e
7. b

Exercise B

1. d
2. g
3. f
4. h
5. a
6. c
7. a

Word Building

1. anacusis
2. neoplasia
3. blepharedema
4. hyperopia
5. audiology
6. corneitis
7. diplopia
8. myringotomy
9. ophthalmoscope
10. retinopathy
11. scleroplasty
12. oculoplasty, ophthalmoplasty
13. otic

Deciphering Terms

1. resembling keratinized tissue
2. new growth
3. abnormal condition of tympanic membrane fungus
4. measurement of the tympanic membrane
5. pertaining to behind the eye
6. paralysis of the eye
7. surgical repair of the ear
8. pertaining to the eye and nose
9. pertaining to the tympanic membrane
10. incision into the cornea
11. drooping of the eyelid
12. movement of the eye
13. pertaining to inside the eye

True or False

1. False
2. True
3. True
4. False
5. False
6. True
7. False
8. False

Fill in the Blank

1. eyes, ears, nose, and throat
2. pupils are equal, round, reactive to light and accommodation
3. astigmatism
4. anacusis
5. presbycusis
6. Meniere's disease
7. glaucoma
8. cataracts
9. diabetic retinopathy
10. macular degeneration
11. hordeolum
12. retinal detachment

Common Diagnostic Tests

1. **Tonometry:** measurement of intraocular pressure
2. **Snellen's eye chart:** vision screening tool that contains rows of letters in decreasing size
3. **Weber's test:** a screening test for hearing that evaluates bone conduction by means of a tuning fork
4. **Rinne's test:** a screening test for hearing that compares bone conduction to air conduction by means of a tuning fork
5. **Audiometric tests:** detailed hearing tests conducted by an audiologist

Multiple Choice

1. a
2. b
3. c
4. a
5. d

Case Study Questions

1. b
2. d
3. d
4. c
5. b
6. a
7. b

INDEX